The
EYE
of the
ARTIST

The
EYE
of the
ARTIST

Michael F. Marmor, M.D.
Professor of Ophthalmology
Stanford University School of Medicine
Affiliate of the Program in Human Biology
Stanford University
Stanford, California

James G. Ravin, M.D.
Clinical Associate Professor
Medical College of Ohio
Surgical Director
Eye Center of Toledo
Toledo, Ohio

*with 190 illustrations
including 120 in full color*

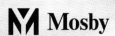 Mosby

St. Louis Baltimore Boston Carlsbad Chicago Naples New York Philadelphia Portland
London Madrid Mexico City Singapore Sydney Tokyo Toronto Wiesbaden

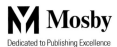

Mosby
Dedicated to Publishing Excellence

**A Times Mirror
Company**

Publisher: Anne S. Patterson
Senior Editor: Laurel Craven
Developmental Editor: Kimberley J. Cox
Project Manager: Linda Clarke
Production Editor: Julie Cullen
Designer: Carolyn O'Brien
Composition Specialists: Christine Poullain, Peggy Hill
Manufacturing Manager: William A. Winneberger, Jr.
Cover art: Rembrandt. *Self-Portrait*. Detail. (The National Gallery, London.
   Reproduced by courtesy of the Trustees.)

Composition by Mosby Electronic Production
Color film by World Color Lanman
Printing/binding by Friesens—Altona, Manitoba, Canada

Mosby–Year Book, Inc.
11830 Westline Industrial Drive
St. Louis, Missouri 63146

Library of Congress Cataloging in Publication Data

Marmor, Michael F., 1941–
        The eye of the artist / Michael F. Marmor, James G. Ravin
        p.   cm.
        Includes bibliographical references and index.
        ISBN 0-8151-7244-3.
        1. Art and visual disorders. I. Ravin, James G. II. Title.
        [DNLM: 1. Visual Perception. 2. Vision Disorders. 3. Famous
        Persons.   WW 105 M352e 1997]
N71.8.M37   1997
704'.08161—dc20
DNLM/DLC   96-27933
for Library of Congress   CIP
97 98 99 00 01 / 9 8 7 6 5 4 3 2 1

CONTRIBUTORS

Christine A. Kenyon, M.A.

Department of the History of Art

University of Michigan

Ann Arbor, Michigan

Philippe Lanthony, M.D.

Centre Hospitalier National d'Ophtalmologie

des Quinze-Vingts

Paris, France

Jody Maxmin, Ph.D.

Associate Professor of Art History and Classics

Department of Art

Stanford University

Stanford, California

Robert A. Weale, D.Sc.

Emeritus Professor

University of London

Senior Research Fellow

King's College London

University of London

University College Hospital Eye Department

London, England

FOREWORD

Paul R. Lichter

Art is a lie that enables us to realize the truth.
Pablo Picasso
The Arts, May 1923

Picasso's statement is as provocative today as it was in 1923. Avant-garde in his words as well as his art, Picasso forced his readers—his viewers—to make an effort to understand the reality of the human experience through the prism of his interpretation. The rewards have been great. And the challenge that this quote presents remains fresh. What is true and what is not true about art?

Because of their particular interest in the mechanics of vision and the more subjective interaction between the eye and the brain, ophthalmologists have long been fascinated with artists, especially in cases where the artist's work has been affected by an ophthalmic disorder. Long asked but still unanswered is the question, "How does the way the eye is made effect our ability to interact with the world?"

As a society we recognize the importance of art and artists. As individuals, we each are moved by art in a very personal way and we wonder at the extraordinary sensitivity of artists, knowing full well that they struggle to deal with life's vicissitudes the same as we. How did Monet work when he was afflicted with cataracts? Did El Greco really have astigmatism, and if so, what was the effect? How was the work of Mary Cassatt influenced by impaired vision? These are just a few of the questions that interest us all.

In *The Eye of the Artist*, Michael Marmor and James Ravin have been good enough to explore these questions for us and provide us with some possible explanations. I have known these two ophthalmologists for many years and have enjoyed following their progress as their ideas evolved from conversation to articles and popular courses at the American Academy of Ophthalmology and finally to this book, which is as beautiful as it is thought-provoking. What the authors and their collaborators have done is to link function (and dysfunction) to art—both the art of the artist and the art of the viewer. The stories of medical disease interest me as a physician, of course, but the issues of how and why art is produced are no less compelling. Although the authors show cases where physiology and disease clearly explain features of art, they also show that most artistic accomplishment is independent of ocular ability (or disability).

Science and art are not mutually exclusive. Each can enhance the appreciation of the other. Such is the accomplishment of this book.

Paul R. Lichter, M.D.
President, American Academy of Ophthalmology
F. Bruce Fralick Professor and Chairman
Department of Ophthalmology, University of Michigan Medical Center
Ann Arbor

FOREWORD

Paul Hayes Tucker

Among the many gifts great artists must possess—from manual dexterity to a capacity for invention—none is perhaps more central to their enterprise than sight. This may go without saying given how essential the eye is to our engagement with the world and to artists' attempts to translate their visual experience into aesthetic forms. But it is surprising how often we forget the significance of sight. From time immemorial, art critics and connoisseurs, when confronted with almost any kind of art, have always tried to define the artist's vision as manifest in the work, referring to the more common, metaphorical sense of the word, just as artists have always been concerned with the powers that produce their personal view of the world or their abilities to realize what they see.

When this most precious of gifts is challenged by accident, age, or human frailty, however, it rightfully becomes a threat of the highest order. In the face of its loss, the value and meaning of this almost magical sense becomes fiercely clear.

Again, this is acutely true for artists. And many of them (surprisingly more than one generally thinks)—Claude Monet, Mary Cassatt, Edgar Degas, Edvard Munch, and Georgia O'Keeffe to name a few—had to face this most terrifying of circumstances and find ways to deal with it. Even Euphronios, one of the most celebrated Greek vase painters of the ancient world, may have suffered from blurred vision when approaching middle age, causing him to abandon painting for pot-making.

The unique collection of essays in this book is a welcome reminder of the multiple battles artists have to wage against a host of visual impairments. As case studies, the essays are both clinical and human, scientific and compassionate. Written by internationally recognized ophthalmologists and their colleagues, they analyze a broad range of physical evidence from artists' writings and personal effects to the recommendations of contemporaneous physicians and the opinions of the artists' friends and relatives as well as the inquiries of art critics and scholars then and now.

Among the essays' many merits is the commendable resistance the authors express to facile associations between medical maladies and artists' styles. This is a happy corrective to the all too frequent explanations for changes in an artist's work as directly related to physical complications. For example, the production of Claude Monet's broadly brushed late *Water Lilies* were interrupted by his cataracts, but their color and form were not necessarily a product of the cataracts.

What such balance permits is what the art itself continually affirms, namely the vitality of the human spirit and the triumph of the aesthetic over the mundane. For despite their difficulties, these artists all managed to rise above their limitations and create works of art of truly lasting power. For that and for these salutary essay, we can be nothing less than grateful.

Paul Hayes Tucker, Ph.D.
Professor of Art
University of Massachusetts
Boston

PREFACE

Michael F. Marmor

My interest in art is of long standing. I was raised in Los Angeles, a leading center for modern art, where my parents (Judd and Katherine) knew many artists and filled our home with beautiful and innovative works. My love of art grew from theirs, as an appreciation of the process and ideas of art as well as the aesthetics. I was also fascinated by science and the intrinsic beauty of mathematics. I majored in mathematics in college, but took as many courses as possible in writing and the humanities; I soon found myself unwilling to give up the humanities for a career in pure science, or abandon science for a career in the humanities. The solution was medicine where science can be applied in a context of human interaction.

During and after medical school I did basic research on the physiology of nerve cells, seeking some seeds of understanding about how the mind works. The retina is an outgrowth of the developing brain, and ophthalmology provided an opportunity to work in neurophysiology (studying the retina and mechanisms of vision) while practicing an enjoyable clinical discipline. My interest in art continued, and soon after joining the medical faculty at Stanford, I took the opportunity to teach (in my spare time) a writing seminar for freshman undergraduates called The Eye and Eyeing. This grew into an upper class course called The Eye and Implications of Vision, which explores the workings of the eye and vision and applies this knowledge to animal behavior and human endeavors such as art, literature, and sport. This course has been given under the mantle of an innovative interdisciplinary major at Stanford called the Program in Human Biology.

From these roots came other invitations to speak or write about eyes and art. Jim Ravin's course at the American Academy of Ophthalmology was so good that I saw no reason to compete in discussing eye disease in artists, so I started a course called Vision and Art to analyze the role of visual function in artistic production and appreciation. This book is in part an outgrowth of our Academy courses, but as a book it reaches beyond an ophthalmologic audience. I hope that our ophthalmologic colleagues will find pleasure in the work, of course, but the principles of vision are universal and the problems faced by artists with eye disease are relevant to anyone interested in art. Understanding vision not only makes the visual aspects of art more comprehensible, but makes it easier to look beyond the purely visual into other realms of art.

This project was motivated, at one point, by the Centennial Committee of the American Academy of Ophthalmology. Jim and I were asked to develop a celebratory volume for the 100th anniversary of the Academy in 1996. Changes in the economics of medicine ultimately prevented the Academy from underwriting the book, which freed us from the need to focus solely on ophthalmology. The book now reflects our broader interests and philosophy about art, medicine, and visual science although we still hope it will honor a century of accomplishment of organized ophthalmology in the United States.

Some special thanks are in order. Jane Marmor has tolerated my late hours with obscure books, excessive phone bills, and aesthetically placed piles of papers in the living room. Her support has been invaluable, and the living room is ready for reclamation. Andrea and David have heard the tale of Mach bands to the point that it is not even an old joke, but they too have provided support and encouragement (and valuable feedback on some of the material). The organizational and secretarial work of Judy Roberts on this book has been only one manifestation of her superlative editorial and administrative skills. Nicole Roberts also helped at a critical phase of the project. Many people have assisted with aspects of the research and with the acquisition of illustrations. Dr. Jan B. Deręgowski invited me to Aberdeen to discuss perspective. Arne Eggum, curator of the Munch Museum in Oslo, kindly provided access to archival material and information; Tomm Skotner helped with translations. Gregory Niemeyer photographed a number of the works and generated contrast and Mach band illusions by computer. Others to whom I am grateful include Dr. Kristina Narfström, Dr. Ellen Bjerkås, Derin Tamyol of Art Resource, Dr. Luisa Orto of Artists Rights Society, and the staff of the Stanford Art Library. Finally, I am grateful to the professional staff at Mosby–Year Book who took on this project and brought it to such an elegant conclusion, especially Laurel Craven, Senior Editor; Kimberley Cox, Developmental Editor; Julie Cullen, Production Editor; and Carolyn O'Brien, Designer.

PREFACE

James G. Ravin

For as long as I can remember, I have been fascinated by the capability of artists to place pigment on a surface and create something interesting. My early memories of large portraits in the corridors of museums remain vivid. I studied at the Toledo Museum of Art as a child and made copies of some of those overwhelming images. As a teenager I took lessons from an artist named Israel Abramofsky, whose works now hang in museums in this country and in France. His experiences in the artistic colonies of Paris and Brittany, and his tales of growing up in czarist Russia were intriguing. He had worked at the Academie Julian in Paris, and he met the artist Paul Signac (whom we describe in chapters 1 and 11) while sketching on the Atlantic seacoast of Brittany. These anecdotes and the paintings remain alive in my mind today, even though I never achieved the standards of these artists in the paintings that I made.

In college I was able to complete nearly all the premedical requirements by the end of my junior year. This permitted me to spend nearly all of my senior year concentrating on the history of art, including a thesis on *art nouveau* glass. When time became available in medical school, I worked with Gerald Hodge, the director of the medical illustration program at the University of Michigan Medical Center. He had access to the back rooms of many museums during a sabbatical spent in Europe, and he had acquired a collection of examples of medical problems illustrated in works of art. We collaborated in writing descriptions of some of these works and published several papers, including articles in the *Journal of the American Medical Association*. Our focus was the subject matter of the works, rather than the artists who had created them. During my residency and later, I turned more toward identifying the problems of artists with physical defects and the effects of these problems on their works. Discussion with colleagues in medicine and in art history about these topics led to requests to speak to various classes and organizations.

At the annual meeting of the American Academy of Ophthalmology in 1980 I gave an overview of the ocular problems of artists to an overflowing room of enthusiastic listeners. Representatives of the Academy felt that this subject would interest the general public, so they publicized it. Soon I was deluged with requests for interviews from the Associated Press, United Press International, and various newspapers. Calls came from television and radio stations all over the United States and abroad. Jane Pauley described portions of the talk on the *Today* show, Paul Harvey discussed the Monet aspect on his radio show, and Charles Kuralt covered it in *On the Road*. Later, reports appeared on the Cable News Network, Public Broadcasting System, in *Art News* and the *New York Times*. After a while, true to Andy Warhol's description of fifteen minutes in the spotlight, things quieted down considerably.

These investigations into the physical problems of artists have interested the public, especially when well known figures, such as the French Impressionists, have been involved. Correlating the correspondence of Monet with his doctors, and describing the effect of cataracts on his work has been interesting. But often working on the cases of lesser known artists has been even more enjoyable because fewer researchers have mined these areas before. Some unsolved challenges remain. What, for example, was Goya's problem? Was it lead poisoning or quinine toxicity? What caused the blindness of two aged French artists, Cheret (the creator of nearly a thousand brilliant posters) and Harpignies (the painter of many idyllic Barbizon landscapes)? Many scholars, physicians, and art historians helped me tie together these studies in a meaningful way. Occasionally, others were not so helpful. I will never forget a conversation about the author and cartoonist, James Thurber, with his ophthalmologist. Knowing the young Thurber had developed sympathetic uveitis after being shot in one eye with an arrow, I wrote and telephoned the ophthalmologist, only to be told that he did not wish to cooperate in discussing the history of a deceased friend. Not every problem ends satisfactorily for the historical researcher. *Sic transit gloria mundi.*

This collection of essays, we sincerely hope, will be interesting and informative to our readers. The capabilities and the limitations of our visual system, our window onto the world, intrigue us all, whether we are trained in art or in science.

Many people merit acknowledgment for their assistance: at the University of Michigan, Department of the History of Art, Professors Diane Kirkpatrick and Marvin Eisenberg; doctoral candidates Christie Kenyon, Nancy Anderson, Pam Reister, Eric Fodor, and Jonathan Perkins; at the University of Toledo, Professor Marc Gerstein; at the Toledo Museum of Art, Leslie Balkany, Larry Nichols, Pat Whitesides, Lee Mooney, and Anne Morris and her staff; and Eddy Mawas, M.D., of Paris. Special thanks to Nancy, Amy, Tracy, and Victoria Ravin.

CONTENTS

INTRODUCTION

THE PROBLEM OF FOCUS

LIGHT VERSUS DARK

ISSUES OF COLOR

PERSPECTIVE AND ILLUSION

The
EYE
of the
ARTIST

Part One

INTRODUCTION

Chapter One

THE EYE AND ART

VISUAL FUNCTION AND EYE DISEASE IN THE CONTEXT OF ART

Michael F. Marmor

Art (in the context of painting and drawing) is fundamentally a visual medium, for both artist and viewer. A few artists have made constructions that are meant to be experienced in darkness or by touch, but in general when we hang art in our homes, travel to cultural or religious sites and visit museums, we expect to *see* art. At the same time, it is obvious that while visual content may be necessary, it is certainly not sufficient to define art. The definition of art depends on issues such as whether or why art differs from design, photography, religion, propaganda, or doodling and how art has meant different things in different ages and to different people. The purpose of this chapter is to focus attention on one aspect of art, vision, which lies at the core of the visual arts no matter how they are defined.

When I say that art is a visual medium, the term "visual" refers to the complex of eye and brain that receives and interprets light and images. Artists don't paint with invisible ultraviolet or infrared pigments, or draw faces that can only be seen with gamma rays. Art is seen by visible light, which is by definition the small portion of electromagnetic radiation to which retinal nerve cells can respond. The way in which our eye and brain recognize and process light is the foundation for how we see. For example, the physical properties and circuitry of retinal cells account for the facts that we see colors during the day but cannot distinguish them by dim moonlight; that the inside of a tunnel appears black as we approach it on a sunny day, while things inside become visible as soon as we enter; that we can read the finest of print and yet be fooled by optical illusions. These are facts of the physics of life and are not options for us (or any artist) to modify or avoid. Artists see the world physically as we all do, although they may be more perceptive than most of us in interpreting the complexity of vision to enhance the impact of their work.

I will review in this chapter characteristics of vision that are relevant to the production and appreciation of art and that represent a substrate for art—sort of tools of the trade. Some of these concepts represent recent advances in our understanding of the visual system, but I hope the medically experienced reader will forgive me for also including some basic material and definitions for readers who lack such background. Information about how the eye works and about eye diseases of artists will not explain art, but to ignore this information is to lose understanding of the constraints that an artist faces in producing a work and that the viewer must face in interpreting a work. Insight into the visual aspects of art is not a threat to artistry; it is rather a means of appreciating better how artistry takes place.

THE VISUAL MACHINE: POWERS AND CONSTRAINTS OF VISION

— STRUCTURE AND OPTICS OF THE EYE —

The eye (Fig. 1-1) is like a camera in that it has a set of lenses in the front (the cornea and the lens) that focus images on a light-sensitive film (the retina) in the back. In the idealized eye, images from far away are perfectly in focus when the focusing muscles are relaxed, and these muscles change the shape of the lens to increase its focusing power and allow us to see objects up close (a process called "accommodation"). In actuality, the human lens is only an instrument for fine tuning our vision; the major focusing element of the eye is the external surface of the cornea. The cornea is more powerful because the power of any lens (whether in the eye or made of glass) relates not only to its shape by to its optical density (i.e., its ability to slow down and bend light) relative to the surrounding medium. There is a big density difference between water and air, so the cornea (which is largely water, like most of the body) is a powerful focusing element; the lens is inside the eye and surrounded by watery fluid of more similar

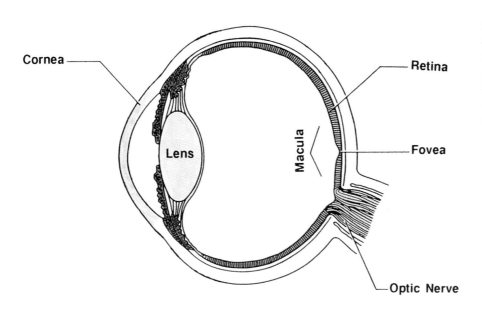

FIGURE 1-1
General structure of the eye. Both cornea and lens focus light onto the retina. The center of vision is at the fovea, which lies within a larger central area called the macula. (*Modified from Goldstein.*[18])

density, so it is much less effective. In a young person, the cornea accounts for roughly three-quarters of the eye's focusing power, and the lens for the last quarter. The importance of the air/lens interface can be especially appreciated under water. You can't see well under water because the density of the water neutralizes most of your cornea's power, and spectacles are useless because glass also has a similar density to water. Fish compensate for the loss of corneal power by having exceptionally powerful lenses (much rounder than ours) within the eye.

The "film" in the ocular camera is a layer of photoreceptor cells in the retina that have evolved the ability to transform light energy into a neural signal. In man, there are two types of photoreceptors, cones and rods, which serve day and night vision respectively. Cones are distributed throughout the retina but are concentrated in a central region called the macula, and they reach a very high density in a small zone called the fovea where they account for good visual acuity as long as there is plenty of light. The cones also are sensitive to color. The rods are sensitive to very dim light but cannot differentiate colors or very fine details. The highest concentration of rods in the retina is just outside the macula, and you may occasionally spot a very dim star that is a little off center, only to find that it disappears when you look right at it (because there are no rods in the very center of the macula). Thus, it is easy to see shapes and movement on a moonlit walk, but one cannot read in the dim light and the world is devoid of colors. In other words, our ocular cameras come automatically equipped with two types of film: a color film with low ASA rating but very fine grain and a black-and-white film with very high ASA rating but coarse grain.

The analogy between eye and camera begins to fail, however, when we look deeper in the retina and at the visual connections beyond. The film in a camera simply records an image, dot by dot, as molecules of pigment are affected by light.

FIGURE   1-2

Simplified diagram of nerve cell layers in the human retina. Visual information must pass through at least two cellular junctions (synapses) before reaching the ganglion cells that form the optic nerve. There are many more photoreceptors than ganglion cells. Sensitivity to contrast comes from the horizontal cells that spread laterally at the level of the photoreceptor-bipolar junctions and exert an inhibitory effect on the bipolar cells. The center of the receptive field for each bipolar and ganglion cell receives excitatory input from overlying photoreceptors, while the larger inhibitory surround represents input from horizontal cells. See also Fig. 1-4. (Modified from Hubel.[1])

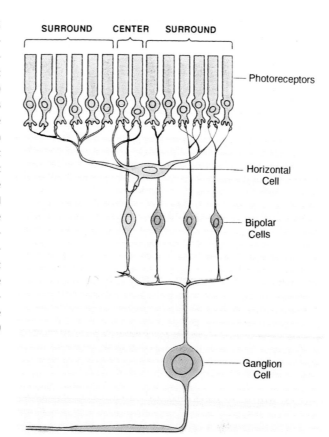

The retina, however, contains several layers of nerve cells that analyze visual information before it ever leaves the eye (Fig. 1-2). The photoreceptors do record the image much like film, but there are roughly 125 million photoreceptors in the eye, and only 1 million fibers in the optic nerve that carries information to the brain. Thus, there is no way that every image imprinted on the photoreceptors can be transferred directly, dot by dot, into the brain; some sort of simplification or coding is required. The nerve cell layers in the retina organize and code the visual image, so that in a very real sense we begin to think about visual images inside the eye. This is not surprising, actually, because the retina develops from an outgrowth of brain tissue in early embryonic life.

Signals from the retina are transmitted via the optic nerve to a way station in the core of the brain called the geniculate body, then to the primary visual cortex at the back of the brain (Fig. 1-3). The extraordinary experiments of David Hubel and Torsten Wiesel, which earned them the Nobel Prize in 1981, showed how visual cortex cells can recognize and sort out specific types of visual information.[1] For example, an individual cortical cell may be sensitive only to the edges of an object oriented in a specific direction and moving in a specific direction at a specific point in space. From the input of hundreds of such cells, which sample each small region in our field of view, the brain can outline and ultimately fill in the shape of everything we see. Furthermore, next to the primary cortex are secondary or association cortices. These regions of the brain are in constant back-and-forth communication with the primary visual cortex, to further refine and interpret the visual information so that we recognize qualities such as texture, movement, and shape.

VISION IS RELATIVE

Why is it so hard to see at dusk, and why does the inside of a tunnel appear so black until we enter it? The answer is *contrast*. In order to codify and simplify images, the retina dwells on comparisons rather than absolutes. In other words, the retina analyzes whether object A is lighter than object B but doesn't worry much about the actual brightness of either object. At first glance this property of vision may seem counterproductive or even poorly designed. But it is actually

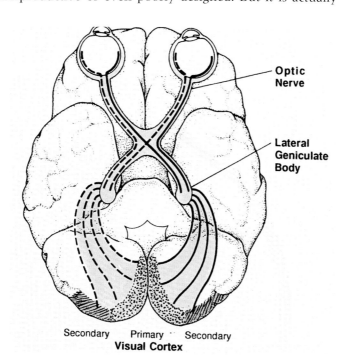

Secondary   Primary   Secondary
Visual Cortex

Optic Nerve

Lateral Geniculate Body

FIGURE 1-3

Visual pathways. Information from the retina segregates in the optic nerve, so the left and right fields of vision are represented by the right and left halves of the brain respectively. *(Modified from Goldstein.[18])*

FIGURE 1-4

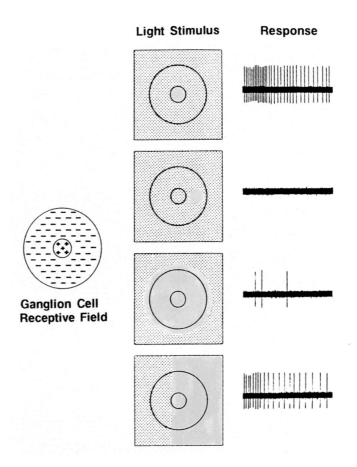

Light Stimulus   **Response**

**Ganglion Cell
Receptive Field**

FIGURE 1-4

Diagram of a ganglion cell receptive field, showing center-surround organization. Light falling in the center excites a vigorous response from the cell, while light in the surround suppresses its activity. Diffuse light over the entire receptive field is only a very weak stimulus because center and surround balance each other. An edge can be a powerful stimulus, however, because only part of the surround is activated when the center is stimulated. *(Modified from Blakemore.[19])*

very useful and in fact critical to normal activity because it allows us to read or recognize the same faces indoors and outdoors, in light or in shadow, even though the amount of light energy reaching our eyes may be thousands of times greater in the bright sun than indoors. Our eyes adjust automatically to these different lighting conditions, much like a modern video camera: in each environment we establish a new scale of grays between black and white. When it is very bright out, the steps between black and white are very large, and anything on the low end (such as a tunnel against the bright sky) will seem pitch black. Once inside the tunnel, however, the brightest lights are in reality rather dim, and the eye quickly establishes a new scale of gray that lets us see where we are going. The reason it is difficult to see at dusk is that everything is gray with little contrast to help the retina make distinctions.

The mechanisms for this contrast sensitivity are hardwired into the retina, as shown in Fig. 1-2. The "bipolar" cells, which bridge between the photoreceptors and the ganglion cells, get input not only from photoreceptors directly before them but also from "horizontal" cells that have long processes which get input from a larger ring of photoreceptors. Horizontal cell synapses have a contrary or inhibitory effect, so each bipolar cell receives a core of positive input from the photoreceptors and, simultaneously, a surrounding doughnut of negative input from the horizontal cells. This "center-surround" organization of the cell's visual input is transmitted to the ganglion cells and then the geniculate body cells. The effects of stimulating the center or the surround alone roughly balance each other, so diffuse bright light, which illuminated both the excitatory center and the inhibitory surround, is *not* a very good stimulus for any of these cells (Fig. 1-4). However, an image with an edge will be a powerful stimulus cell since the edge

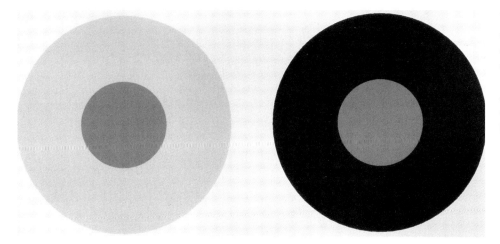

FIGURE   1-5

A contrast illusion. The central circles appear to differ in brightness but are actually identical (see Fig. 1-6). The light background makes the gray appear dark by contrast, while the dark background makes it appear light.

can stimulate the center strongly while only partially activating the surround (thus leaving a net positive effect). Because of this neural circuitry, our retinas are exquisitely sensitive to contrasts between light and dark, but they are relatively insensitive to the absolute brightness or dimness of the world around us.

These hardwired properties of vision account for many optical illusions. For example, when you look at the two gray circles in Fig. 1-5, it appears that the one on the left is much lighter than the one on the right. However, connecting the central gray zones (Fig. 1-6) reveals their cores to be identical. Why does this occur? Because our retinal circuitry is powerfully stimulated by the contrast between white and gray, which tells our brain that the gray is "dark" (or between black and gray, which tells the brain that gray is "light"), while the circuits are poorly equipped for judging the absolute brightness of each gray center.

An extension of this concept is the interesting phenomenon of Mach bands, which can be found in many types of art[2] and in the world at large (see Chapter 6). A Mach band is the illusion that at a sharp junction between light and dark, images appear a little brighter on the light side and a little darker on the dark side. As a consequence the gray rectangles in Fig. 1-7 appear to be graded or fluted, although each one is actually an even shade of gray. Conversely, if an artist draws a junction that accentuates lightness and darkness, viewers will have the illusion that *everything* to one side is lighter than on the other side (Fig. 1-8). Other examples are shown in Chapter 6 (see Figs. 6-1 and 6-2). This technique has been used very effectively in Asian brush paintings to make some areas (such as sky) show contrast with others (such as mountains or moon) (Fig. 1-9; see also Fig. 6-4). On the other hand, Renoir carefully blurred the edges of faces and arms to eliminate contrast and thereby create a sense of softness. A modern artist who used Mach bands rather explicitly was the early-twentieth-century American Arthur Dove, whose small but richly colored works explored new aspects of visual imagery. Mach bands have appeared intentionally or unintentionally throughout the history of art, and their power comes from the fact that their effects on the eyes and brain are intrinsic to neural structure and thus impossible to avoid even with a rational knowledge of what is going on.

—   THE MEANING OF COLOR   —

Color is recognized and interpreted at several levels within the retina and brain. It is initially perceived by the cone photoreceptors which are most concentrated in the central vision area of the retina. There are three types of cones, each containing a different pigment so that it is sensitive to a specific range of the color

FIGURE 1-6

The illusion of Fig. 1-5 with the central gray zones connected to show that they are identical.

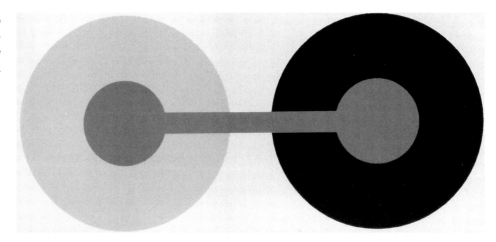

FIGURE 1-7

Mach bands. Illusionary bands of light and dark appear at each junction because of the contrast between the different regions of gray. The net effect is that each gray region appears shaded from dark to light, whereas they are all evenly colored. Mask the junctions to prove this to yourself. Understanding that the mechanism of this phenomenon resides in the center-surround organization of the bipolar cells does not make it any less powerful visually.

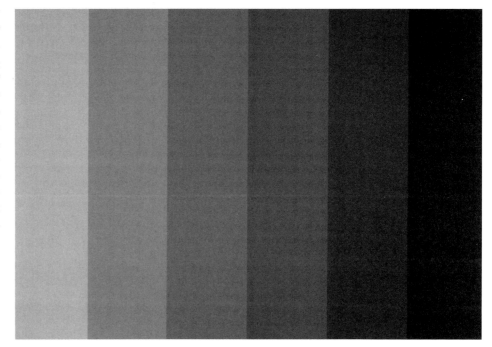

spectrum (red, green, or blue, as in Fig. 1-10). When we look at a colored object, our cone photoreceptors sample the relative amounts of red, green, and blue light and these proportions define the color.

The three types of cone photoreceptors account for the initial recognition of color, but the retina still must code this information (just as it does black and white information) so that it can be conveyed to the brain through a limited number of optic nerve fibers. The fundamental code is the same: the retinal cells are wired to recognize contrast. In the case of colors, the cells respond most vigorously to contrasts between reds and greens or contrasts between blues and yellows. It is conceivable (although not proven) that this may influence subjective sensations that are common to most people. For example, reds and greens are colors that do not blend well for most of us, and when juxtaposed they seem vibrant or even disturbing while other combinations, such as red and yellow, seem much more harmonious. These dynamic sensations have been exploited by Anuszkiewicz and other "optical artists" (Fig. 1-11; see also Figs. 13-5 and 13-11).

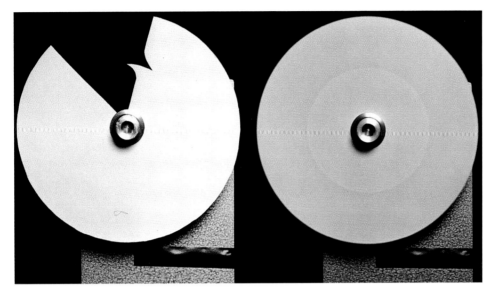

Illusory brightness difference on a spinning disc produced by Mach bands between two evenly shaded regions (Craik-O'Brien effect). The stationary disc (*left*) shows a wedge pattern that one might think would produce simply a band of light and dark between two equally gray zones. In the photograph of the spinning disc (*right*), however, the outer circle appears darker because of the Mach band: the eye recognizes the light-dark contrast, but not the gradual recovery, so everything on one side of the junction is seen as light and on the other side as dark.

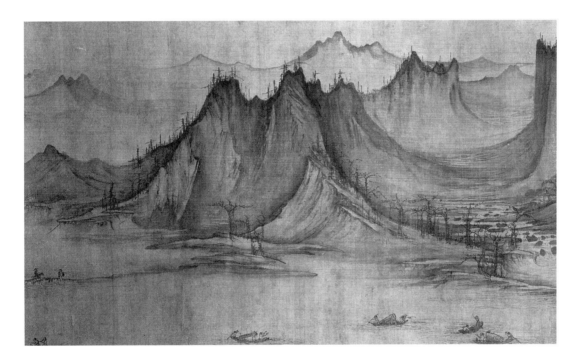

The eye is exquisitely sensitive to color differences and is much more acute in discriminating between colors, and recognizing their relationship to each other, than it is in judging the absolute color of the environment. In fact, the brain uses the constancy of relationships to maintain recognition of colors in faces, clothes, and other patterns even when the color of the background lighting varies (such as at sunset or in the colored lights of a disco). Contrast in color perception is easy to demonstrate to yourself (Fig. 1-12). When you stare for a period of time at a strongly colored object, your eyes become adapted (and thus relatively less sensitive to that color); if you then look at a white page, you will see an afterimage in the complementary colors (e.g., red for green). Similarly, an object *next* to an area of color will appear to take on the complementary color. This can lead to striking illusions, as in Fig. 1-13 where X patterns (of equal color) appear blue and pink respectively because of different backgrounds.

FIGURE 1-9

Hsu Tao-ning. c. 970-1051/1052.
Fisherman's Evening Song.
Detail. Handscroll; ink on silk c. 1049. The mountains are outlined with Mach bands which make them appear dark. However, parts of the mountains in the foreground are no darker than the stream, and the center of those in the background matches the sky. (*The Nelson-Atkins Museum of Art, Kansas City, Missouri [Purchase: Nelson Trust].*)

FIGURE 1-10

Spectral sensitivity of the three types of human cone photoreceptors. The visible spectrum of electromagnetic energy (i.e., light) ranges from about 400 nanometers (blue) to 700 nanometers (red). Individual cones are most sensitive to blue, green, or red light.

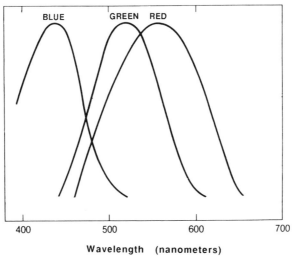

FIGURE 1-11

Anuszkiewicz. *Plus Reversed.* Oil, 1960. The jarring effect of this painting is enhanced by the juxtaposition of red and green, colors that oppose each other in the circuitry of the retina and brain. *(©1996 Richard Anuszkiewicz/Licensed by VAGA, New York, NY. Archer M. Huntington Art Gallery, The University of Texas at Austin. Gift of Mari and James A Michener, 1991. Photo credit: George Holmes.)*

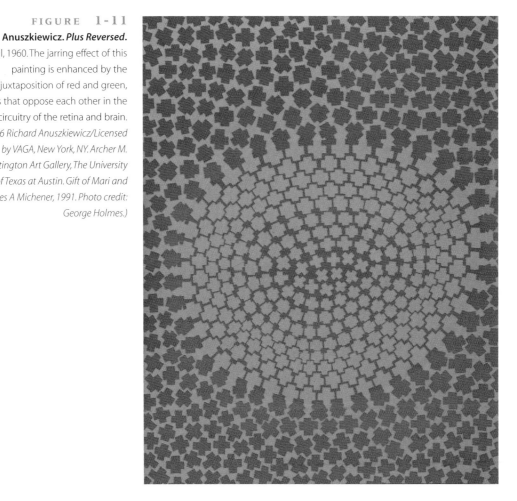

A further complexity of color perception is the fact that our ability to see colors depends in part on the size of the objects being viewed. This occurs because each individual nerve cell in the retina and brain perceives a finite (albeit small) part of the world. If adjacent dots of color are tiny enough, they will fall entirely within the input to single photoreceptors or single ganglion cells, and the eye cannot dis-

FIGURE 1-12
Complementary afterimages. Look at the dot between the four colored rectangles for 30 seconds. Then look at the dot on the white background and you will observe rectangles of complementary colors (green for red, yellow for blue, etc.).

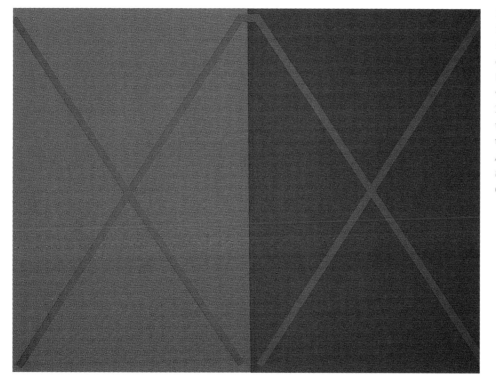

FIGURE 1-13
Study in reversed grounds. This plate shows an illusion of simultaneous contrast. The X pattern surrounded by pink appears falsely blue and vice versa, although one can see that the X patterns have identical color where they join at the top. Cover this junction to strengthen the illusion. *(From Albers J: Interaction of Color [Plate VI-3, top], © Yale University Press, New Haven, Conn., 1963.)*

criminate between them. It is this principle that lets us see smooth halftone pictures in a magazine or colors on a television screen. These images are both composed of dots having only three or four colors, but the dots are too small to resolve so the colors blend according to physical laws for the mixing of colored paint or light respectively (Fig. 1-14). Superimposing two colored lights will add brightness and give the color perception of an intermediate wavelength, whereas paints or pigments are light-absorptive (subtractive) media. Light is absorbed by pigment, and the color we see represents only those wavelengths that are *not* absorbed, that is, those that pass through or are reflected. Thus, mixing red and green paint yields

FIGURE   1-14

Additive and subtractive color mixtures. Mixing light is additive, since each new light adds energy. The combination of red and green is brighter than either alone and is perceived as yellow. Mixing paint is subtractive, since paint appears to have a color only because it absorbs other wavelengths. Mixing red and green paints yields a dark and murky brown.

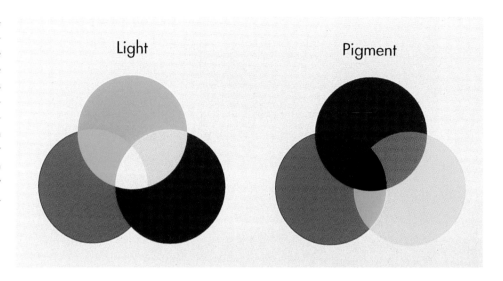

FIGURE   1-15

Signac. *Entrance to the Grand Canal, Venice.*

Oil, 1905. These spots of color are large enough to appear vibrant through contrast between them (rather than blend as do the tinier dots in pointillist works). Compare with the paintings by Seurat illustrated in Chapter 11. *(The Toledo Museum of Art, Toledo, Ohio; Purchased with funds from the Libbey Endowment, Gift of Edward Drummond Libbey. ©1996 Artists Rights Society (ARS), New York/SPADEM, Paris.)*

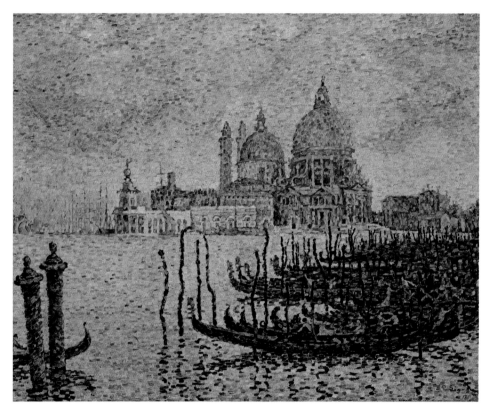

a murky brown pigment, but when the red and green light of adjacent pixels is intermixed on a television screen we see a bright yellow. This effect is not appreciated in magazine illustrations because the ink dots in color printing are not discrete; they overlap to a large degree and mix like paints rather than light.

As you may surmise, our perception of color in an image made up of dots will change if the size of the dots increases to the point that retinal cells can recognize the individual dots and the contrast between them. Under these conditions, colors that juxtapose will appear bright and vibrant rather than mixed. In some of Seurat's "pointillist" paintings, there are areas where he juxtaposed dots of relatively complementary colors; these areas seem bright when viewed up close but

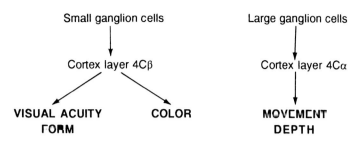

PARALLEL VISUAL PATHWAYS

	VISUAL ACUITY FORM	COLOR	MOVEMENT DEPTH
Light requirement	High	High	Low
Resolution	Small	Medium	Large
Contrast sensitivity	Low	Low	High
Response speed	Slow	Slow	Fast

FIGURE 1-16

Parallel pathways within the visual system for fine resolution, color perception, and depth and motion.

become curiously pale and gray when viewed from far away where the dots are no longer discernible individually (see Chapter 11).[3] For this reason, some of the neo-Impressionists, like Signac, preferred "divisionism" in which larger spots of color are used to produce a more vibrant appearance (Fig. 1-15).

THE BRAIN AND PARALLEL SYSTEMS OF PERCEPTION

The mechanisms described so far serve to get images into the visual system, but there is a large jump between recording a shape on the visual pigments of the retina and recognizing what that object may be. The visual system represents a series of way stations, at each of which information is further categorized and refined. However, components of visual information such as resolution, form, color, dynamic structure, and movement are kept relatively independent as they travel through the visual system until they reach the secondary or association visual cortices of the brain (Fig. 1-16).[4,5] Here there is crosstalk between the components so that our conscious perception integrates all aspects of vision.

This segregation of components of vision begins within the retina. We have already noted that rods and cones divide the tasks of night vision and day vision respectively, and that the cones initiate the process of discriminating colors. By the time this information reaches the ganglion cells, the last set of retinal neurons, the cells have become further specialized. Smaller ganglion cells carry information about color or about fine spatial discriminations and resolution; larger ganglion cells concern themselves primarily with motion recognition and spatial orientation.

These divisions are maintained at the first visual way station, the lateral geniculate body, which lies deep in the core of the brain, and the output from the geniculate body segregates to different layers within the primary visual cortex (see Fig. 1-3). Our image of the world (field of view) is mapped topographically onto the visual cortex in such a way that the bulk of the cortical area corresponds to the central core of our visual field where we have good acuity. Each square millimeter of visual cortex surface samples one small area of the world, giving information about edges, colors, movement, and so on. The individual cortical cells can be quite specialized, and most respond only to select stimuli such as a bar of light oriented at a particular angle to the horizon and sometimes moving only in

FIGURE   1-17
Directional sensitivity of cortical cells.
The excitatory part of the receptive
field for the cell on the left is a bar of
light oriented vertically, and even a
slight tilt makes the stimulus ineffec-
tive. Nearby cells will be sensitive to a
slightly different direction, so each
small region of cortex samples a full
range of directions. More complex
cortical cells, like the one on the
right, require not only proper orientation of the stimulus but also movement in a particular direction.
(Modified from Blakemore.19)

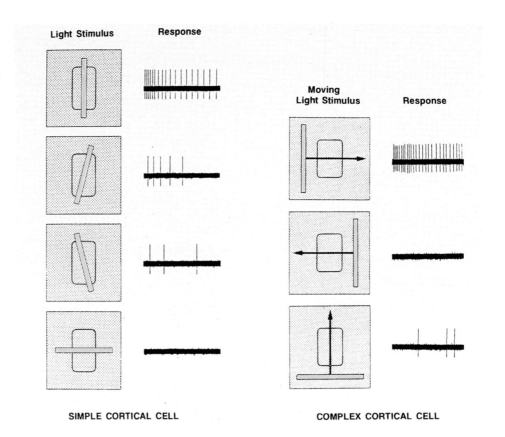

a particular direction or having a particular length (Fig. 1-17). Our visual awareness of shapes is derived from hundreds or thousands of such cells responding primarily to the edges of objects. However, even this sophisticated mapping of the
visual world is not sufficient to explain how we recognize and interpret the more
subtle characteristics of vision such as texture and speed of movement.

Some of this further refinement of visual understanding takes place in nearby
areas of brain called the visual association cortices (see Fig. 1-3). The primary visual cortex is labeled V1 in anatomic classifications, and the visual association areas
are V2, V3, V4, V5, and so on. Largely through the work of Dr. S.M. Zeki,[5] we
know that the V1 map of the visual world gets transferred to the various association areas, but in a selective way. Thus, area V3 receives color-free information
relating to form and motion, and this area is primarily concerned with the delin-
eation of dynamic form. Area V4 specifically receives color-coded information and
serves as a key element in the assignation of color to images. Area V5 is specialized
for movement and is the area that helps us to recognize the directionality and speed
of motion of objects within our view and appreciate the sensations of kinetic art.[6]

Illusory phenomena reinforce the idea that different aspects of visual perception are processed in parallel through the visual system.[4] For example, one can
compose a picture on a television monitor of red dots on a green background and
make the object move on the screen. This movement will appear to fade or cease
if the intensity of the colors are adjusted to be equally bright for the movement-
sensitive cells. Because these cells cannot tell the difference between red and
green of equal intensity, they are unable to register the motion of the figure. A
related phenomenon in art, discussed by Dr. Margaret Livingstone,[7] is illustrated
in Fig. 1-18. The beauty of this Matisse is captivating, but on inspection it is obvious that the colors spread rather far beyond the various outlines of the figure and
objects. Why isn't this sloppiness terribly bothersome to us? Possibly because our

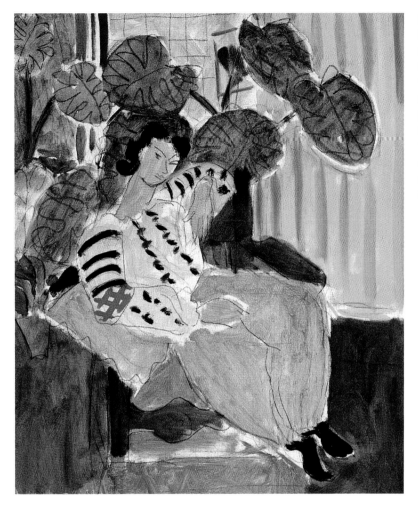

color perception system is not geared to the recognition of sharp outlines, and thus we can accept the clear discrimination of the outlined shapes from our form and resolution pathways while also accepting the general awareness of color, so our first conscious impression is of a normally colored image.

Parallel visual pathways also govern the interaction of contrast, spot size, and color that modulate our perception of pointillist and divisionist paintings. We noted earlier that colors juxtaposed as tiny dots blend according to the laws of mixing lights, but there is more to the story. Different cellular pathways in the visual system serve color perception and the resolution of small objects or shapes. The system that recognizes fine print and tiny dots does not respond to color, while the system that recognizes color cannot discriminate very small lines or objects. Thus, you may notice as you walk back and forth in front of a pointillist painting that there are three different ranges of perception: up very close, the colored dots are discrete objects; at middle distances, the colors blend (since the dots are too small for the color pathway to discriminate), but one still recognizes that the painting is stippled with the high-acuity pathway; far away, both colors and dots blend imperceptibly. As Lanthony argues in Chapter 11, these perceptions are intrinsic to the power of these paintings.

As powerful as these parallel pathways may be, there is also ample evidence that they are not totally independent and that the different visual cortical association areas interact with each other. Even equiluminant colored dots can be seen to move under the right conditions, suggesting that separation of processing sys-

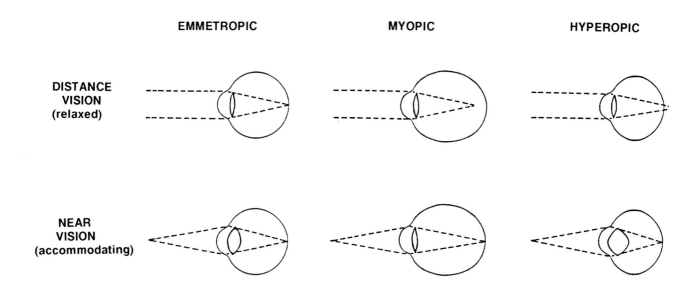

FIGURE 1-19
Diagrams of the optics of the human eye. In an ideal (emmetropic) eye that is fully relaxed, objects at infinity are perfectly focused on the retina. A nearsighted (myopic) eye is too long under these conditions, while a far-sighted (hyperopic) eye is too short. Thus, a myopic individual will need less (and a hyperopic individual more) accommodation than normal to focus on close objects. (The differences in eye size and in lens thickness with accommodation have been exaggerated in these diagrams.)

tems for color and motion is not absolute. The concept of parallel processing of resolution, form, color, depth, and motion within the brain is a useful framework to describe aspects of our vision, but it is also a simplification because our brain ultimately intertwines all of these perceptual processes to interpret what we see.

EYE DISEASE AND THE ARTIST

The working of a normal eye puts certain constraints on vision, as we have noted, and abnormalities of the eye or disease will further complicate the processes of vision. This section is a brief introduction to eye diseases that are particularly relevant to art and artists.[8]

— ALTERED FOCUS —

Although the relaxed idealized eye is perfectly in focus for objects at infinity, many of us have eyes that are not ideal. A myopic (nearsighted) eye is too long relative to its lens system, so that faraway images come to a focus in front of the retina and appear blurred (Fig. 1-19). Objects very close can be seen clearly because the rays of light diverging from them move the point of focus farther back on the retina. Myopia is easily corrected with spectacles or contact lenses that have a concave shape.

A hyperopic (farsighted eye) is too short for its lens system, so faraway objects come to a focus behind the retina (Fig. 1-19). Such an individual must focus or accommodate, even to see faraway objects and must focus additionally in order to read. Hyperopia is corrected with convex lenses.

Some eyes also have a degree of astigmatism, which means that the surface of the eye is slightly barrel shaped rather than spherical. In other words, images are focused more strongly in one direction than another. This can be corrected with glasses that are ground to compensate for the asymmetry or with hard contact lenses that have a spherical outer surface. Most soft contact lenses that mold to the surface of the eye do not correct astigmatism.

An optical problem that affects virtually all of us eventually is "presbyopia," the loss of accommodation with aging (see Chapter 2). As we get older, the lens becomes less elastic, and, as a result, we lose the ability to focus over the whole

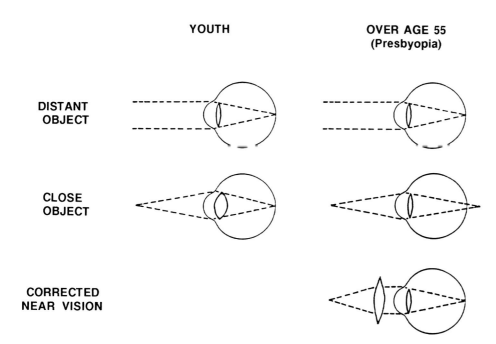

YOUTH   **OVER AGE 55**
(Presbyopia)

DISTANT OBJECT

CLOSE OBJECT

CORRECTED NEAR VISION

FIGURE 1-20
Diagrams showing the loss of accommodation with age (presbyopia) in an emmetropic eye. Distance vision is unchanged, but after age 55 the lens is no longer able to change its shape sufficiently to accommodate for near objects. A convex reading lens compensates for the lost accommodation. (The magnitude of lens change are exaggerated in this diagram.)

range from infinity to near (Fig. 1-20). By age 50, most people who see clearly at distance are no longer able to read comfortably with the same correction, and convex lens power is prescribed for reading (to be added to whatever one wears for distance). It is important to understand that presbyopia is only a problem with *range* of focus; it is not ordinarily accompanied by any change in preexisting myopia or hyperopia. Older individuals do not usually change their distance correction; they simply cannot focus over as broad a range as when they were young.

How do these refractive errors affect artists? They must have been critical in ancient times, when no glasses were available to correct poor vision. It is doubtful that any nearsighted individuals painted landscapes in ancient Egypt or that any severe hyperopes entered service as a fine jeweler. There is actually some evidence that presbyopia may have modified the artistic career of one of the most famous vase painters in ancient Greece, as discussed in Chapter 5.

Writers have speculated about whether the fuzzy appearance of the world to uncorrected myopic eyes may have influenced the Impressionists as they explored new ways of painting. Some of the Impressionists may have been myopic, but glasses were available when they needed or wanted them. Monet's early works were representational and very precise, which either disproves he was myopic or confirms his use of spectacles. Renoir was probably not very myopic, as discussed in Chapter 3, and his misty figures (Fig. 1-21) derive from a conscious blurring of border contrast rather than poor acuity (see Chapter 6). Myopia might have given ideas to some Impressionists, but they had the capability of seeing clearly when they wished, so their artistic choices must have come from the intellect and soul rather than being forced on them by their eyes.

Could presbyopia have played a role in the changing styles of painters such as Rembrandt (Fig. 1-22), whose painting became coarser and less precise as he aged? (See Chapter 2.) I am doubtful of this, for several reasons. The changes in Rembrandt's style were gradual and continued over many years rather than occurring abruptly at presbyopic age. His drawings include a picture of Titia, his wife's older sister, doing close work with glasses (Fig. 1-23), so that spectacles were clearly available and familiar to Rembrandt. It is difficult to ascribe changes in artistic style to refractive changes unless an artist has complained about visual

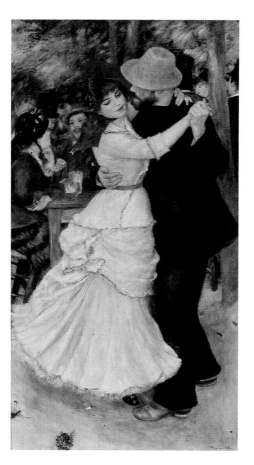

FIGURE 1-21
Renoir. *Dance at Bougival.*
Oil, 1883. For a detail showing how Renoir achieved the soft misty appearance of his figures, see Figure 6-11. (*Picture Fund. Courtesy, Museum of Fine Arts, Boston.*)

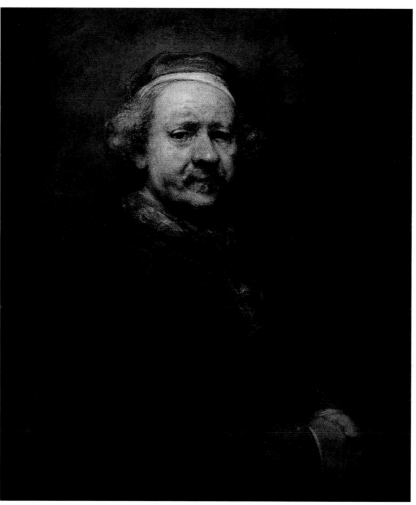

FIGURE 1-22
Rembrandt. *Self-Portrait.*
1669. This portrait was painted when the artist was in his early 60s. (*The National Gallery, London. Reproduced by courtesy of the Trustees.*)

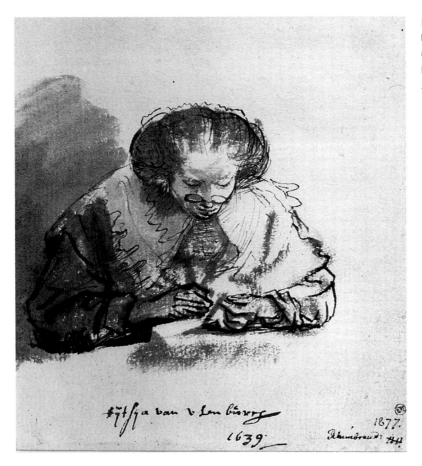

FIGURE 1-23
Rembrandt. *Portrait of Titia van Uylenburgh.*
Drawing, 1639. (*National Museum, Stockholm.*)

problems or the changes are so striking as to be unequivocal. Could this be the case with respect to astigmatism, which by its nature distorts the world in one axis and compresses it along another? For example, are the elongated figures in El Greco's paintings the result of an uncorrected astigmatic error? (Spectacles were available in El Greco's day but not with astigmatic correction.) This argument fails for several reasons, as discussed in Chapter 4.

—— COLOR DEFICIENCY ——

The red-sensitive and green-sensitive pigments in cone photoreceptors are inherited through genes on the X chromosome (the sex chromosome). Since males have only one X chromosome (the other is a Y), men who have an abnormal X will be unable to make the usual distinctions between red and green colors (Fig. 1-24). This is a very common problem, and roughly 10% of men in the United States have some degree of altered sensitivity to reds or greens. For most color-deficient men the problem is mild and may never be noticed except with very pale or dark colors, but a small percentage of men cannot distinguish bright orange-red from bright green.

Abnormal color discrimination would clearly put an artist at a disadvantage, at least insofar as that artist wished to paint in colors. Artists may well be unaware of a mild abnormality, and its effects would be hard for viewers to discern given allowances for individualism and style. At least two well-known artists had a recognized severe color deficiency: the French engraver Charles Meryon (see Chapter 9) and the art deco sculptor Paul Manship. Both realized their problem as young men and switched to artistic forms that did not utilize color. A red-green color-

FIGURE 1-24

Reduction of a color-test plate showing a pinkish "8" against a green background. Individuals with red-green color deficiency have trouble distinguishing the more orange-colored dots from green and see a "3" instead. (The test colors may not be accurate in this printing. For visual testing only the original plates should be used.) *(From Ishihara.[20])*

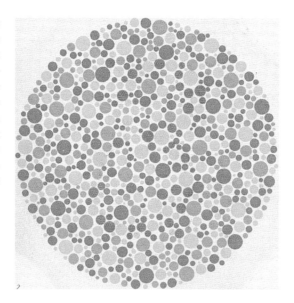

deficient artist might produce pictures like Meryon's early pastel (see Fig. 9-4) which lacks color diversity and is dominated by yellow and blue.[9] A severely color-deficient artist, painting from an unmarked palette, might also make gross confusions between certain colors such as orange and green or purple and blue-green. Manship's son related that his father "was painting a still life with a brown jug when [a colleague] asked him why he had painted the jug green. Paul defended himself by invoking artistic license, but in fact he had thought that he was matching the jug's true color. For a painter, color blindness is obviously a severe handicap, but for a sculptor it might prove an advantage: the eye, not being distracted by color, could concentrate on form."[10] This latter is a romantic notion, because most color-deficient people do see colors—they just don't see the same array as everyone else. Nevertheless, it is said the military has at times used red-green deficient men to spot camouflage, with the idea that they will be less influenced by color and thus more sensitive to recognize differences in brightness or texture that would differentiate a camouflage covering from the surrounding environment.

Even if we speculate that some well-known painters are likely (on statistical grounds) to have had at least mild color deficiency without knowing it, it is hard to guess who they are or to judge the extent that this problem influenced their work. There has been discussion,[8] for example, as to whether the great English landscape painter Constable was color deficient because of his emphasis on greenish and yellow tones and his spare use of reds. I doubt we will ever know for sure, but many of these characteristics are also found in the works of other artists of the same period, and Constable painted a number of pictures with accurate rainbows (Fig. 1-25).

It is particularly difficult to separate color style from necessity in retrospect, because artists are aware not only of what they see but of what they are expected to see. It is common knowledge that grass is green, and an artist may reach for a green-labeled tube of paint without necessarily perceiving the color in a normal manner. For example, Monet complained bitterly that colors were fading as his cataracts grew dense (see the discussion on cataracts in this chapter; see also Chapter 15), but he learned to compensate. In 1918, while struggling to work on his great water lily canvases, he told a visitor, "If I have regained my sense of color in the large canvases I've just shown you, it is because I have adapted my working methods to my eyesight and because most of the time I have laid the color down haphazardly, on the one hand trusting solely to the labels on my tubes of paint and, on the other hand, to force of habit, to the way in which I have always laid out my materials on my palette."[11]

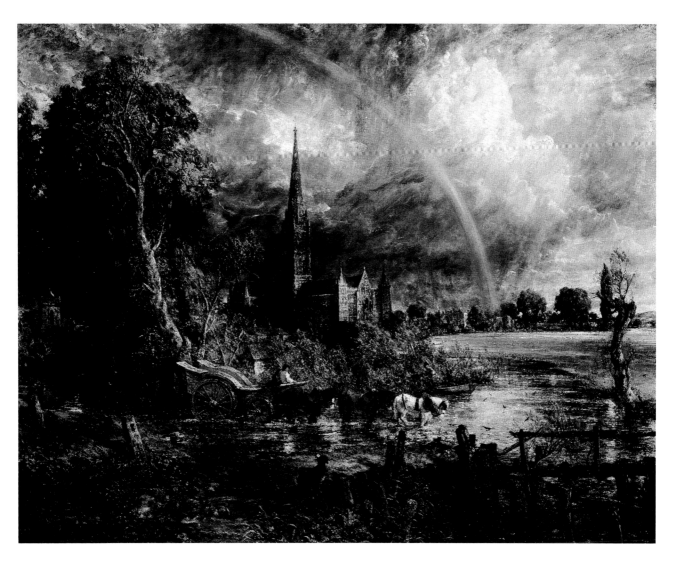

Another example of this dilemma is the case of Fernand Léger. There are notes in the literature that he may have been color deficient, and even though there are documentary reasons to discount this assertion,[12] the case illustrates again the difficulties of retrospective analysis. Léger used strong unmodulated colors in his paintings (Fig. 1-26), and in retrospect one cannot tell if they were chosen by observation or name. However, it is highly doubtful that Léger was color deficient. In his writings, he spoke frequently about the pleasures of different hues, and he worked with strong colors by choice and not necessity: "It was about 1910 that Delaunay and I began to liberate pure color in space. . . . Color was free; it had become a new reality."[13] Furthermore, his widow who had worked with him for 32 years never noticed any abnormalities in his color vision.[14]

FIGURE 1-25

Constable. *Salisbury Cathedral from the Meadows.*

1831. *(On loan to The National Gallery, London.)*

--- CATARACTS ---

The human lens lays down new tissue throughout life, and as we age it becomes less elastic, more dense, and slightly more yellowish. In most people, these changes are subtle and do not affect visual acuity, except for the development of presbyopia (see earlier in this chapter) that necessitates reading glasses or bifocals. In some people, however, the lens becomes so sufficiently opaque that vision is compromised; then we call it a cataract. In modern society, cataracts are rarely a major visual problem, because surgery to remove them is highly success-

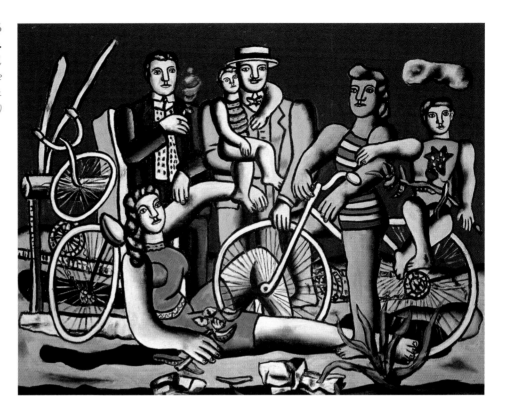

ful and the cataract can be replaced with a plastic lens implant inside the eye. However, cataract surgery was dangerous and only marginally successful in ancient times, and as late as the first part of the twentieth century it was still fraught with complications. Even when it was successful, thick and uncomfortable spectacles were required postoperatively.

We don't know which artists in ancient times had their careers shortened by the development of cataract. None is specifically recorded to my knowledge, but it is highly likely that some who lived long lives would have been afflicted. In more modern times, we do know of several artists whose career was shortened or modified by the development of cataract. The most notable and well-studied example is that of Claude Monet, the great French Impressionist, as evident in Fig. 1-27 and detailed in Chapter 14. Mary Cassatt also developed cataracts in her older years and stopped painting as a result, even though she had surgery on one eye (see Chapter 15). Other painters who have had cataracts late in life include Honoré Daumier and Marsden Hartley.

The changes in color perception that occur with cataract surgery are intriguing. As a cataractous lens becomes more yellow, a person will see a progressively more yellow world and lose particularly the brightness of blue (since it is absorbed by yellowish pigment). This is evident in some of Monet's paintings before his cataract surgery (Fig. 1-27; see also Chapter 14). However, a drift toward yellowish and reddish tones is not by itself a reliable indicator of early cataract in painters (see Chapter 2). For example, some have speculated that Turner might have had cataracts as a cause of his yellowish impressionistic scenes such as *Mortlake Terrace* (Fig. 1-28). However, he painted in this style over many years (he lived almost 25 years after painting *Mortlake Terrace*), which would be unlikely if cataracts were progressing, and even his later works (see Figs. 8-3, 8-4, and 8-5) often contained points of exquisite detail that are inconsistent with a dense cataract.

The issue is further complicated by the facts that painters may know from their palette what colors to use and that some artists may seek to paint what they

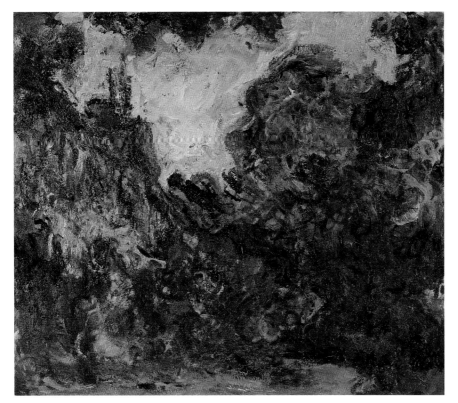

FIGURE 1-27

Monet. *House at Giverny.*

Oil, 1922. The subject is barely recognizable in this canvas, painted within a year of Monet's cataract operation. *(Musée Marmottan, Paris. © Musée Marmottan.)*

remember of a scene (rather than what it looks like through their cataract). In this latter case, a painter might use more, rather than less, intense blue to produce an image that overcomes the yellowness of the lens and restores the remembered blueness of sky or water. An example of this effect is shown in Fig. 1-29. The artist was a woman with cataracts under the care of Dr. G. Karpe in Sweden. After Dr. Karpe removed her cataract, she called the picture "horrible" and "too blue" and gave it to the hospital.[15] When cataracts are removed, patients often note an immediate brightening of colors because the hazy filter is no longer present. It is said that blues often become darker and brighter postoperatively, but some patients may perceive yellows to be brighter (perhaps because they now can be better discriminated from other colors).

— OTHER DISEASES —

Many diseases can affect the eye, of course, and being an artist does not make one immune to them. Some eye conditions are not related directly to vision, such as blockage of the tear ducts (which bothered Pissarro; see Chapter 16) or the loss of only one eye to a tumor (as happened to Joshua Reynolds).[16] Conditions that affect vision primarily, such as bilateral disease of the retina or the optic nerve, cannot help but affect an artist's work.

Degas complained of poor vision much of his life and had a central blind spot in the better of his two eyes, which annoyed him continually. Nevertheless, he compensated for this problem and painted in spite of it—although his pictures seem to become coarser with age and he shifted progressively to sculpture as his vision became worse. The cause of his disease remains unproven, although some interesting hypotheses have been raised (see Chapter 17). Another painter with intrinsic eye disease was Edvard Munch, most famous for his haunting image, *The Scream.* He suffered hemorrhaging inside one eye at age 66, and as his vision

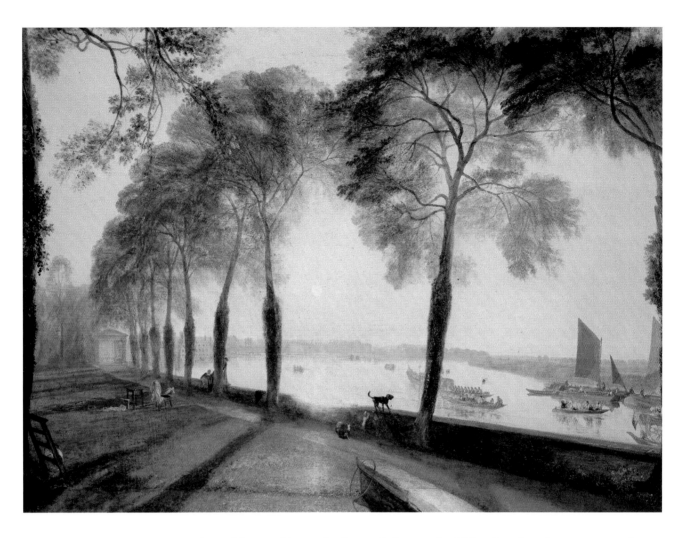

cleared he could see shadows of the residual blood within his eye. Munch put images of these floaters into paintings (see Chapter 18). Wyndham Lewis lost his sight from a pituitary tumor that pressed on his optic nerves, and he painted his last picture with the aid of a magnifying glass.[17] James Thurber, famous for his wistful cartoons as well as his humorous essays, had poor vision all of his life as a result of a childhood injury. His brother accidentally shot an arrow into his right eye, which was lost, and the left one developed "sympathetic" inflammation. The disease smoldered for years. By his 40s, Thurber could only draw on a huge easel, and he ceased drawing in his early 50s.

CONCLUSIONS

Art is a grand enterprise of the human spirit, and it is not explicable on the basis of how the eye works anymore than it is explicable solely on the basis of politics, religion, historical convention, or esthetic mores. It represents a combination of these influences, and it distills the quirks of the artist and viewer, the biases of upbringing, the politics of propaganda, the vagaries of religion, and probably many other factors as well. Understanding these influences adds to our appreciation of art, for it helps us to understand what motivated an artist and why certain conventions of presentation are used. Similarly, understanding how

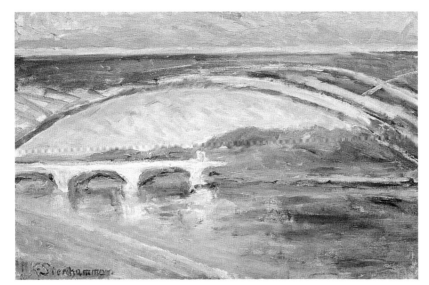

FIGURE   1-29

Painting made by an artist with cataracts. She apparently added blue to compensate for lost sensitivity through the aged lens, because after surgery she thought the picture was too blue. *(Reproduced courtesy of Peep Algvere, MD)*

our eye responds biologically to images can add to our appreciation of how colors, contrast, and other visual elements contribute to (or may modify) an artist's intentions or results. For the most part, the eye should be an unseen tool for the appreciation of art, but an awareness of how vision works can help us to see many aspects of art with a fresh eye.

— REFERENCES —

1. Hubel DH: *Eye, Brain and Vision*, Scientific American Library, New York, 1988.
2. Ratliff F: *Contour and contrast, Sci Am* 226:90-101, 1972.
3. Ratliff F: *Paul Signac and Color in Neo-Impressionism*, Rockefeller University Press, New York, 1992.
4. Livingstone M, Hubel D: Segregation of form, color, movement, and depth: Anatomy, physiology, and perception, *Science* 240:740-749, 1988.
5. Zeki SM: *A Vision of the Brain*, Blackwell, Oxford, 1993.
6. Zeki SM: The neurology of kinetic art, *Brain* 117:607-636, 1994.
7. Livingstone MS: Art, illusion and the visual system, *Sci Am* 258:78-85, 1988.
8. Trevor-Roper P: *The World through Blunted Sight*, Thames and Hudson, London, 1970 (rev ed: Allen Lane, London, 1988).
9. Lanthony P: Daltonisme et peinture, *J Fr Ophtalmol* 5, 6-7:373-385, 1982; Lanthony P: Dyschromatopsies et art pictural, *J Fr Ophtalmol* 14, 8-9:510-519,1991.
10. Manship J: *Paul Manship*, Abbeville Press, New York, 1989, p. 15.
11. Thiebault-Sisson F: Les nympheas de Claude Monet, *Revue de l'Art Ancien et Moderne* 52:41-52, 1927. Translated and reprinted in CF Stuckey (ed): *Claude Monet 1840-1926*, Art Institute of Chicago, Chicago, 1995, p. 248.
12. P. Trevor-Roper described Léger as color deficient in an early article (The influence of eye disease on pictorial art, *Proc Roy Soc Med* 52:721-744, 1959), but he later felt uncertain about the reference and left it out of his book.[8] Trevor-Roper's original source was an article in German by J Strebel (Prolegomena optica zum bildnerischen Kunstschaffen, *Klin Monatsbl Augenheilk* 91:258-272, 1933), but the relevant passages describe a painter, "G.E." (Maler G.E.), rather than Léger.
13. Léger F: *Functions of Painting*, Viking Press, New York, 1973, p. 150.
14. Larsson S: *Konstnärens Öga*, Natur och Kultur, Stockholm, 1965, pp. 63-64.
15. Anecdote related by Peep Algvere, MD, of St. Erik's Eye Hospital, Stockholm.
16. Weiss ET, Davidorf FH: The medical history of Sir Joshua Reynolds and the enucleation controversy, *Ophthalmic Forum* 1:63-64, 1983.
17. Michel W: *Wyndham Lewis*, University of California Press, Los Angeles, 1971.
18. Goldstein EB: *Sensation and Perception*, ed 3, Wadsworth, Belmont, Calif, 1989.
19. Blakemore C: The baffled brain. In RL Gregory, EH Gombrich (eds): *Illusion in Nature and Art*, Charles Scribner's Sons, New York, 1973, pp. 9-47.
20. Ishihara S: *Tests for Colour-Blindness*, Kanehara Shuppan, Tokyo, 1995.

Chapter Two

AGE AND ART

Robert A. Weale

Bernard Levin, the well-known, long-sentence-writing columnist of the *London Times* once commented on the extensive lives granted by Providence to orchestral conductors. It did not take a great deal of statistics to demonstrate that their life expectancy was similar to the norm. This point is worth making because artists have likewise been credited with a greater-than-average longevity, with Titian who may have reached his 90s being cited as a typical example rather than as an exception. One faces the question of whether artists, surely subject to the same biological processes of senescence as the rest of us, betray their years in their style, their technique, or their handling of whatever medium they may be using. There are several reasons for asking this.

On the mechanical side, the decline of muscular prowess would be expected to have an impact on an artist's sculpture and carving; in painting and graphic arts, there may be effects on the precision with which fine brush strokes are executed or with which a needle is guided across a copperplate in preparation for the etching process. In this context, it is perhaps possible to distinguish between relatively fine and coarser work. Michelangelo would work on marble into his 80s, but the surface of the *Holy Family* in Santa Maria dei Fiori, one of his last works, is none the worse for this.

A similar argument applies to Bernini who also lived into his 80s and likewise preserved his extraordinary manual dexterity into these later years (witness the delicate Apollo and Daphne in the Villa Borghese in Rome, dating from 1615, and the baldachin in St. Peter's in Rome, completed some 50 years later). Not too much evidence for an artist's biological age should, however, be looked for in his artifacts: it is always possible that he destroyed what to him appeared to be failures (see Chapter 14) or, if they turned out to be unsatisfactory from a commercial point of view precisely because they showed signs of decline, they may have been hidden from public view.

The situation is clearer when it comes to painting. We have a great deal of information on aging processes of the visual apparatus. True, observations on several painterly features, supposedly related to senescence, are based on correlation and may sometimes be confused with stylistic peculiarities. On the whole, however, certain characteristics relating to brushwork and the use of color occur repeatedly in artifacts produced by older painters, and, while proof may not be possible, an explanation in terms of biological changes seems highly plausible. The following is intended not to be an exposition of detailed changes in the ocular visual and perceptual system[1] but rather a sketch which will enable us to examine whether an artist's work betrays his age.

PRESBYOPIA

By far the best known visual correlate with age is the need for reading glasses. The normal human visual system has evolved for distant objects to be focused on the retina without any muscular effort on the part of the eye. Such an eye is called emmetropic. When the gaze is directed to a nearby object, for instance, no farther in distance than 4 or 5 meters, such an optical system would give rise to an out-of-focus image being formed on the retina; the nearer the object the greater the distance between the image plane and the retina and, hence, the greater the resultant blur.

This disparity has been eliminated in the human eye by the evolution of accommodation, or the ability of the lens of the eye to change its power. In effect, it becomes thicker the nearer the object viewed. In young eyes, the mechanism underlying accommodation is involuntary and involves the activity of the ciliary muscle and, probably indirectly, the muscles of the iris (the latter effect is thought to be different in monkey and man, even though both are primate species).

However, even children can exhibit a progressive decline in the reflex ability of the lens to adjust to distance. The decline continues monotonically throughout the first 4 or 5 decades of life and becomes symptomatic in temperate countries after the age of 40. The condition is then referred to as presbyopia. The condition used to be attributed to a sclerosis, or hardening, of the lens, a hypothesis that has been successfully undermined during the last 30 or so years. The underlying causes have recently been reexamined,[2] and the condition has been related to more modern ideas than is done in the run-of-the-mill textbooks: presbyopia appears to be associated not only with aging but also, for example, with the progressive growth of the lens and the resulting change in its suspension. The need for reading glasses occurs when symptoms are experienced by virtue of close print becoming illegible.

Note the above use of the word "reading." Conventionally, reading matter is kept at a distance of some 30 to 40 centimeters, and, if the lenses cannot accommodate to this distance, then a reading correction of 2.5 to 3.0 diopters will be needed for the formation of an in-focus retinal image. But artists who paint or model do so at almost twice reading distance: manipulation, let alone the inter-

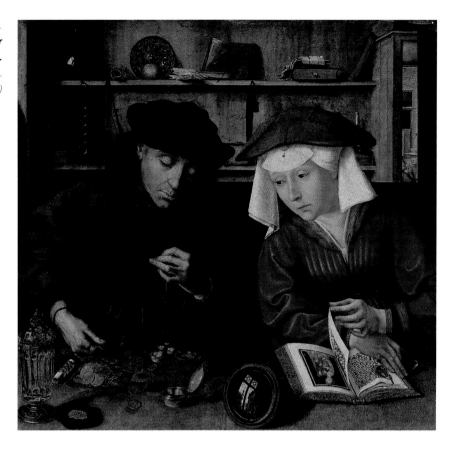

vention of brushes, would be awkward at the closer distance. Evidently, then, the correction needed for readers is inapplicable for those using their eyes at a greater working distance, as is true also, for example, of musicians.

This means that whereas the majority of presbyopes can manage with one type of reading glasses or bifocals, older musicians and artists are likely to need two, namely a reading and a working pair. In theory, painters may manage also with just one type, but one must remember that work does not involve just focusing the eyes but also tilting one's head, and this may create considerable discomfort with polyfocal corrections, as users of computer monitors will be only too ready to confirm.

The wearing of an appropriate correction provides an adequate operational solution for older artists rendering a scene occupying no more than approximately one plane beyond their easel. Thus, even as presbyopes will they be enabled to continue with portraiture, with painting from memory, and with landscapes. However, a rapid variation in near frontal planes could be problematic: still lifes or close table scenes such as *A Money Changer and His Wife* by the Flemish artist Quentin Massys (Fig. 2-1) are hardly topics for painters who are "getting on." When painting this panel, the artist was 47 or 48 years old.

A practical manifestation of senescence among classical artists is provided by their brushwork. The heartless designation of a coarsened stroke, referred to in Rembrandt's case by the most delicate Italian word "impasto" is one such result. Compare the brushwork in Rembrandt's *Saskia*, painted in his 30s, with his *Jewish Bride*, which dates from his 60s (see Fig. 1-22 for a self-portrait painted late in his life). In itself, this change can be attributed to presbyopia alone only if other putative causes can be excluded. And this is difficult, because it could be a matter of stylistic development or, alternatively, stem from what follows.

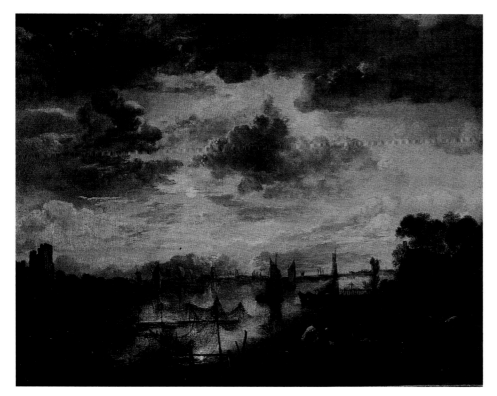

FIGURE 2-2

van der Neer. *Fishing by Moonlight.*

c. 1665-1669. Kunsthistorisches
*(Museum, Vienna, Austria. Erich
Lessing/Art Resource, NY.)*

CONTRAST VISION AND FINE DETAIL

There is a close link between the ability of the eye to resolve fine detail in an object and the perceived contrast of the detail against its background. In general, the finer the detail the greater the contrast needed to render it visible. Plainly we cannot read in very dim surroundings, though we may be able to pick out a tree. From this point of view, we can appreciate how unrealistic has been the rendering of moonlit scenes by some artists. For example, the seventeenth-century Dutch artist Van der Neer in effect converted a colorful sunlit, high-contrast waterscape into a colorless moonlit high-contrast painting (Fig. 2-2), in which nets, small branches, and distant masts are easy to discern. While he was clearly aware of the fact that colors need lots of light for them to stimulate the color-mediating cones (see Chapter 1) and that they vanish in dim light, he had not appreciated that this is also true of fine detail. He was not alone in this respect, for Stechow refers to a moonlit landscape by the older artist Massys, saying that "it is not much more than a daylight landscape plus a nice nocturnal sky,"[3] a way, incidentally, in which the Japanese artist Utagawa Toyoharu rendered a nocturnal naval battle scene even in the nineteenth century.

With advancing years, the ability to resolve fine detail diminishes no matter how high the contrast. The deterioration does not occur for coarse detail, and the explanation may well lie in the fact that even newborn babies have an ability to recognize, and therefore to perceive, relatively large features such as the details of the maternal face. The ability to process fine detail is acquired only well after birth. It would seem therefore that what comes last goes first. It is worth mentioning in this connection that Rembrandt appears to have given up the demanding art of etching in his early 60s whereas he continued to paint until the last year of his life. Also noteworthy is that in not one of his 30 or so self-portraits does he show himself wearing glasses; his penetrating studies make it unlikely that his later self-portraits were masked by personal vanity. Glasses were clearly admissible in a portrait and appeared in Gerard Dou's painting *Rembrandt's Mother*.

A variety of factors may contribute to this decline in contrast sensitivity. Some may be purely optical. The pupil diameter diminishes systematically with age, and a very small pupil is optically less efficient than one, say, 3 millimeters in diameter. Again, the clarity of the lens may become slightly impaired even in the absence of what might be referred to clinically as a cataract, that is, a decrease in lenticular transparency causing a measurable reduction in visual acuity.

Other contributing factors may involve the nervous retina by virtue of losses of receptors; intermediate cell stations, such as bipolar cells; and changes in the brain itself. For example, it has been shown that myelin, the fatty substance that allows the white line of Gennari, or the striate area of the visual cortex, to be distinguished from the gray matter is lost progressively with age. Its function is presumably to minimize crosstalk between various elements: if its concentration drops, spatial detail conveyed in cortical messages may become indistinct, leading to a blurred perception.

It follows, therefore, that an artist's declining rendering of fine detail, as correlated with age, is hard to pin down to any specific cause.

COLOR

The use of color in paintings is classically based on the ability of the eye to match one color to another. The artist sees a blue sky and mixes pigments, say, ultramarine and a touch of leaf-green and lead-white, to mimic the appearance of the sky. The match may be deliberately "off" to convey mood or to achieve a contrast with some other important object, but, in essence, there is an example of what Gombrich[4] has called "matching and making." The pigments are matched to the original surface colors, and the painting is then produced.

There are several conditions, however, that may inadvertently frustrate a match. One results from a color defect, usually a genetic condition, dealt with in Chapter 1. This manifests as an underuse of the palette in that a small number of pigments appear to match a larger number of object colors: a red sea may be literally so because the eye fails to distinguish between red and green.

But, insofar as aging is concerned, the principal effect on the rendering of colors may be exerted by the lens of the eye. We have already encountered its potentially nefarious influence in the reference to presbyopia, when it is liable to lead to a degradation of the retinal image and therefore to a painting matching it. Another age-related effect relates to the coloration of the lens. Right from birth, it yellows systematically, and it progressively absorbs more and more blue and violet light rays. This increase in absorbance is independent of the appearance of haze, mentioned earlier, and appears to be a normal, nonpathological phenomenon. It is evident that, to the extent to which blue and violet rays are absorbed by the lens, they cannot reach the retina and therefore fail to contribute to the perception of color: what cannot be seen cannot be matched and therefore cannot be made.

If the so-called cooler parts of the visible spectrum are attenuated by the aging lens, then matching will be dominated by the complementary warmer tones, and paintings will look predominantly ocher or brownish. A typical example of this is Titian's *Apollo and Daphne*, which, even after old and discolored layers of varnish had been removed, presents with brownish overtones. Rembrandt offers other examples, and, in more modern times, a similar trend can be observed in the

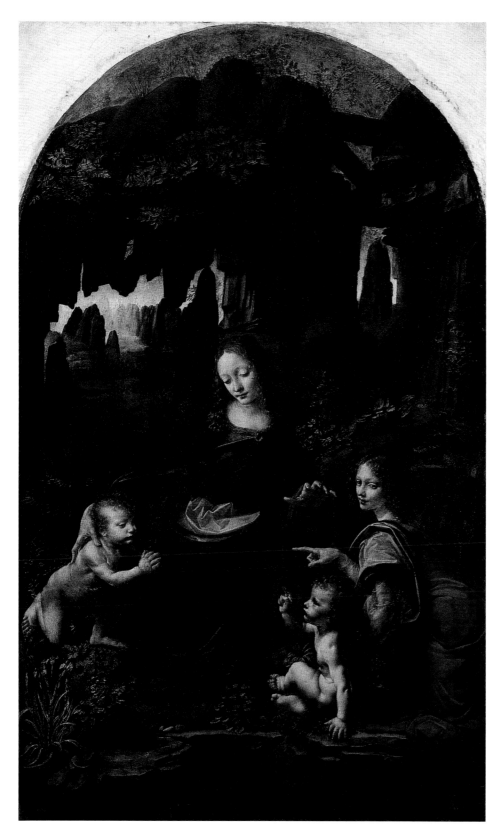

FIGURE   2-4
Leonardo. *The Virgin of the Rocks.*
c. 1503. *(National Gallery, London.)*

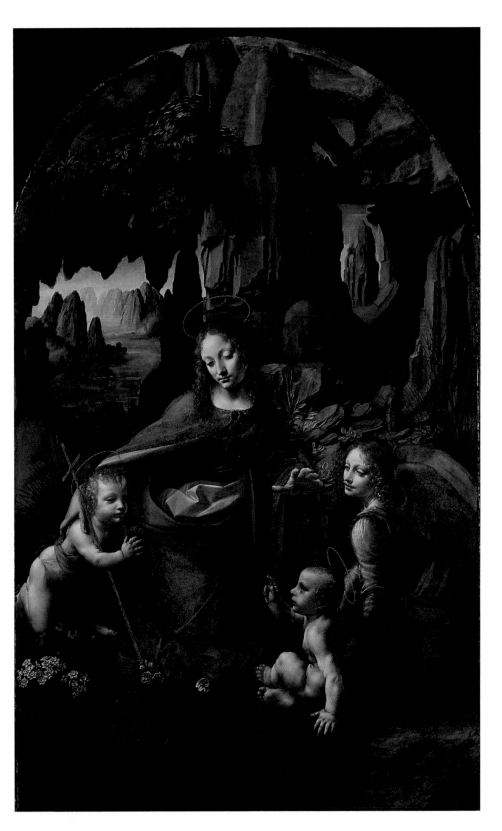

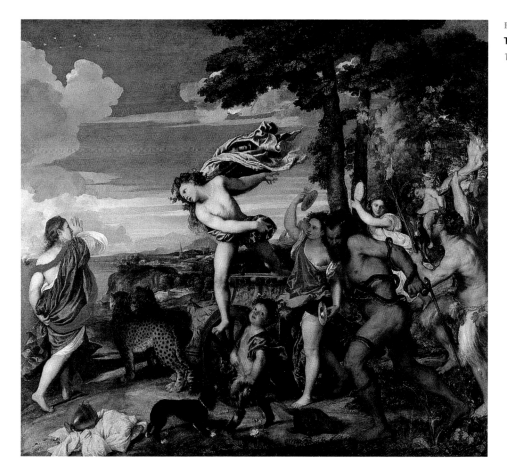

FIGURE   2-5

Titian. *Bacchus and Ariadne.*

1520. (National Gallery, London.)

work of the early-twentieth-century French artist Rouault. It is, or course, possible for an artist to disguise this potential change in tonality: if he relies on memory or reflexes, he will paint a sky blue because he knows that it is blue, not because this is how it appears to him. Psychologists distinguish between memory colors and matched ones, a subject more amenable to laboratory experimentation than to an application in stylistic analysis.

One of the most intriguing examples of memory colors, however, is found in two paintings by Leonardo. They present the same theme, both titled *The Virgin of the Rocks*. One version is in the Louvre, the other in the National Gallery in London. The earlier Louvre work was painted when Leonardo was 32 years old, the other some 20 years later (Figs 2-3 and 2-4). There are important stylistic differences between the two versions, the later of which has probably been modified by the De Predis brothers. The later Christ Child is drawn in an inferior manner; there are halos where the first version shows none; the London painting shows a diminished notion of depth, and the detail is coarsened in more than one place. However, the overriding difference is to be found in the use of color.

John Shearman[5] has attributed the difference in chromatic tonality to the possibility that the earlier version was seen in daylight, whereas the later one was meant to convey lunar lighting. This is possible, but one cannot rule out the notion that the coloration is the result of Leonardo developing a cataract. It has been suggested that he was a myope,[6] and myopia is a risk factor for nuclear cataract. Now it might be argued that an internal lens filter might not affect painting, much as a hypothetical astigmatism cannot explain El Greco's Mannerist

FIGURE   2-6
**Titian. *Christ Crowned
with Thorns.***
c. 1570. *(Alte Pinakothek, Munich,
Germany. Scala/Art Resource, NY.)*

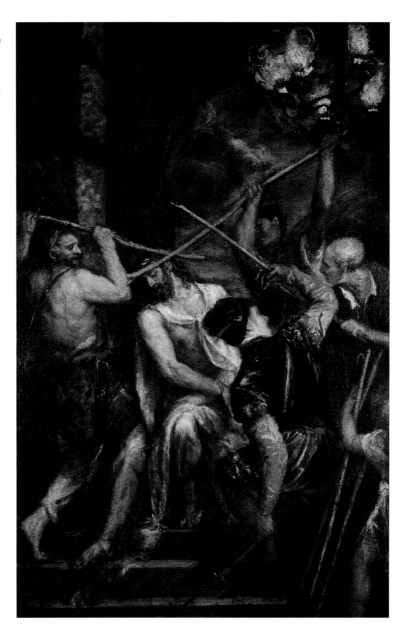

elongations. If a scene is viewed and painted through a filter, the effect of the latter should be negligible. This will be true only if the filter does not affect color recognition to such an extent as to cause confusion in a spectral range where a young eye would detect differences. Moreover, only one version of *The Virgin of the Rocks* could have been painted from life. Even if the earlier one was based on models, the later one must represent a memory painting, so the question of matching pigment mixtures to surface colors does not arise.

A strong argument against the cataract hypothesis is the loss of red in the angel's garb on the right in the late version, which would not be expected if such a textile were viewed through a yellow lens filter. However, a point in support of the influence of a possible cataract in Leonardo's eyes is the degradation of the Virgin's conventionally blue cloak and the overall loss of detail in the second version as a whole. If the Virgin's cloak were to be seen in moonlight, as suggested by Shearman, its color would admittedly appear desaturated, but its luminous tonality would be relatively high because the rods in our eyes, which operate at low light levels, are relatively more sensitive to the blue part of the spectrum than is true of the daylight cones.

However, in the final analysis, when advancing hypotheses about Leonardo's eyesight based on the appearance of his works, one skates on thin ice. The reason is that he was an inveterate experimenter with pigments—which is why *The Last Supper* decayed to a disastrous state even during his lifetime—and, if some pigments change faster than others, the tonal balance of paintings is going to be modified. Even standard pigments become more transparent over the centuries so that underpaintings (in Italian, *pentimenti*) become visible.

There are fewer problems in this respect in connection with Titian's oeuvre. The brilliant blue of the sky and the pizzicato detail in his *Bacchus and Ariadne* (Fig. 2-5) can be compared with the broadened strokes and the browned coloration in the Munich *Christ Crowned with Thorns* (Fig. 2-6), of which it was said that "no painter before Titian had ever attempted to convey the lack of precision which characterises the vision of the aged." A juxtaposition of these two works illustrates, but does not prove, what might be expected on the basis of what we know about ocular aging.

To summarize, a survey of the output of a number of artists in relation to their age may lead us to think that what we see is only to be expected. But we should never forget that paint and varnishes age, too. While the latter may be removed and replaced, often to accompanying screams of disapproval from the antagonists of "cleaning," the senescence of pigments is much slower than that of man but equally irreversible. If two factors change in tandem, a hypothetical single underlying cause, such as the artist's changing eyesight, is hard to pin down. We are condemned to almost idle speculation, for what may pass as a sign of ocular change may equally validly reflect a change in style.

── **REFERENCES** ──

1. Weale RA: *The Senescence of Human Vision*, Oxford University Press, Oxford, 1992.
2. Pierscionek BK, Weale RA: Presbyopia—a maverick of human aging, *Arch Geront Geriatr* 20:229-240, 1995.
3. Stechow W: *Dutch Landscape Painting of the Seventeenth Century*, Phaidon, London, 1966, p. 173.
4. Gombrich E: *Art and Illusion*, Phaidon, London, 1960.
5. Shearman J: Leonardo's colour and chiaroscuro, *Z Kunstgesch* 25:13-47, 1962.
6. Weale R: Leonardo and the eye, *Doc Ophthalmol* 68:19-34, 1988.
7. Fernau J: *An Encyclopaedia of Old Masters*, Thames and Hudson, London, 1958, p. 299.

Part Two

THE PROBLEM
OF FOCUS

Chapter Three

RENOIR'S MALADIES

THE MEDICAL TRIBULATIONS OF AN IMPRESSIONIST

James G. Ravin

The paintings of Pierre-Auguste Renoir (1841-1919) are works of sensual pleasure, not of the intellect. In describing his efforts, Renoir said, "When I look at the old masters I feel a simple little man, yet I believe that among my works there will be enough to assure me a place in the French School, that school which I love so much, which is so pretty, so clear, such good company."[1] There is no doubt that he succeeded. Renoir is of interest medically. His health was adversely affected by a severely disabling case of rheumatoid arthritis, and alterations in his eyesight may have affected his artistic production.

RENOIR'S HEALTH

The first notable medical event to affect Renoir's method of work was a bicycle accident in 1880. He broke his right arm, but being ambidextrous he began to paint with his left arm. In a letter, he treated this jocularly: "I am enjoying working with my left hand, it is very amusing and it's even better than what I would do with the right. I think it was a good thing to have broken my arm, it made me make some progress."[2]

In December 1888 Renoir was afflicted with his first serious bout of rheumatoid arthritis, the illness that was to cause him much grief in the years to come. In addition to the arthritis, he was also having problems with his eyes, ears, and teeth.

Rheumatoid arthritis gave him massive deformities of multiple joints and reduced his ability to use his hands. Many photographs of the artist during his last decades of life show his arthritis. Motion pictures of Renoir painting still exist, and even if we take into account the jerky motions of early cinematography, he is seen jabbing at the canvas, rather than painting with a smooth motion. The arthritis certainly reduced his manual dexterity. He lost the ability to make fine motions with his fingertips and tended to move the brush with his forearm and arm, which caused broader and less detailed depiction of forms (Fig. 3-1). One biographer felt that this had a great impact on the evolution of his style: "Because of his illness, Renoir was never able to regain the heights of genius, diversity, and innovation apparent in his greatest paintings of 1872 through 1883. Nonetheless, despite what could have been regarded as a devastating incapacity, the heroic Renoir was able to cope with and transcend his illness by sustained creative work. In this light, the paintings of his last 30 years are courageous and, toward the end, miraculous."[3]

As his arthritis worsened, Renoir found the extremes of temperature in Paris more and more uncomfortable, and he spent more time in the south of France. To others, he appeared timid and frail. In 1897 he had another bicycle accident, refracturing his right arm. As in 1880, he turned to painting with his left arm. Pissarro, the elder statesman of French Impressionism, complimented him, saying, "Didn't Renoir, when he broke his right arm, do some ravishing paintings with his left hand?"[4]

Julie Manet frequently visited Renoir and wrote that "Renoir's health changes every day, sometimes he looks fine, but then his feet and hands swell; this disease is really very annoying, and he, so nervous, puts up with it with a lot of patience. . . . It is so painful to see him in the morning not having the strength to turn a doorknob."[5]

Medical treatment for Renoir's arthritis included oral antipyrine (an anti-inflammatory drug similar to aspirin), sunshine, walks, massage, baths, purges, application of heat, and visits to spas such as Aix-les-Bains. A surgeon frequently scraped at his rheumatoid nodules. Despite a good appetite, he lost weight and was only 97 pounds in 1904. He used a cane but later had to be transported in a wheel-

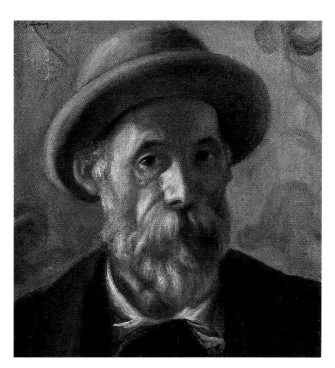

FIGURE 3-1
Renoir. *Self-Portrait.*
Oil on canvas, c. 1899. (© *Sterling and Francine Clark Art Institute, Williamstown, Massachusetts.*)

chair or a portable chair. His son Jean described his appearance at age 70: "What struck outsiders coming into his presence for the first time were his eyes and hands. His eyes were light brown, verging on yellow. His eyesight was very keen. Often he would point out to us on the horizon a bird of prey flying over the valley. . . . As for their expression, imagine a mixture of irony and tenderness, of joking and sensuality. . . . His hands were terribly deformed. Rheumatism had cracked the joints, bending the thumb toward the palm and the other fingers toward the wrist. Visitors who weren't used to it couldn't take their eyes off this mutilation. Their reaction, which they didn't dare express, was: 'It's not possible. With those hands, he can't paint these pictures.'"[6] He became unable to pick up objects. Photographs show linen strips or bandages in an x-shaped pattern over his hands, which have been misinterpreted as straps to hold the brush in his hands. Actually, the cloth served as a dressing to protect his fragile skin from damage by the wooden brush. He became unable to change brushes, and an assistant did this for him.

In 1912 he suffered a stroke but recovered within a few months. During his last few years, arthritis crippled him so badly that he remained confined to his room for weeks at a time. Although extremely thin and severely arthritic, he painted until his death at age 78 in 1919.

FIGURE   3-2

Renoir. *Vines at Cagnes.*

Oil on canvas, c. 1908. *(The Brooklyn Museum. Gift of Colonel and Mrs. E.W. Garbisch.)*

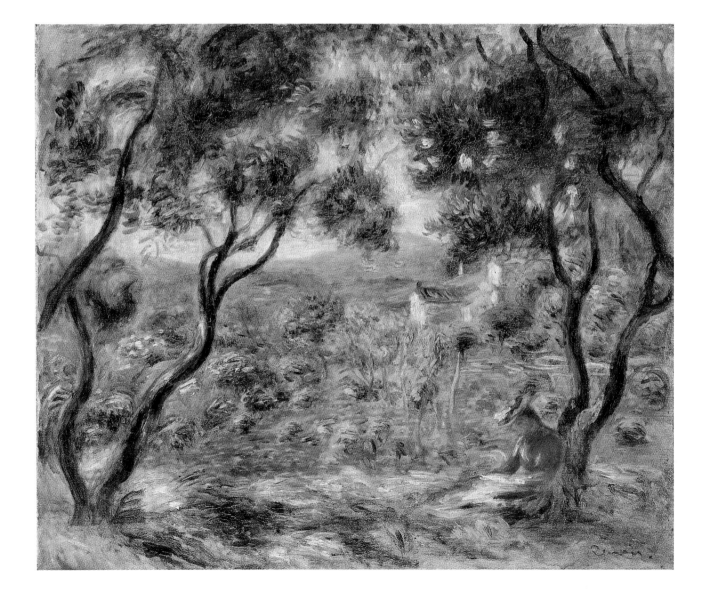

AGE-RELATED STYLISTIC CHANGES

In his late works (Fig. 3-2) Renoir changed his style, painting with less detail and with a marked preponderance of warm, rich, red tones. He was working in the warm sunlight of southern France at the time and preferred to use warm colors so that if they darkened with time, the warmth would still be apparent.[7]

It is possible that these changes are due in part to alterations in his eyesight. Our ability to see details and perceive color changes with age (see Chapter 2).

Renoir's canvases reveal a change from a wide range of hues in his early works to late paintings in which reds predominate. Similar changes in details and colors with advancing age are found in the works of other artists, notably Titian, Constable, Rembrandt and Rouault.[8,9] Changes in color perception can be explained by the fact that the ocular media, especially the lens, act as a yellow filter to block transmission of some light rays on their way to the retina. The result is that a disproportionate amount of violet, blue, and green light rays are filtered out, while red and brown are relatively unaffected.

MYOPIA OR PRESBYOPIA?

Was Renoir nearsighted? Trevor-Roper, in *The World through Blunted Sight*[10] says yes, but I have not been able to confirm this in any other reference to the artist. Trevor-Roper wrote, "Renoir,…according to his biographer Vollard, when looking at pictures would step back a few paces [in other words out of his limited near-range of clear vision] in order to give it the effect of an Impressionistic picture." Of course, this statement does not prove Renoir was myopic. It indicates he liked to look at his paintings from a certain distance, just as many myopic as well as nonmyopic artists often do. Trevor-Roper continues, "He was then 60; and even at 64, when none of us who are not myopic can expect to read at near range without convex spectacles, he liked to examine petit-point close to, taking it in his hands." This misinterprets Vollard, for Vollard was not referring to a form of embroidery but rather to pointillism, the method of painting devised by Seurat to cover the canvas in small spots of color. Trevor-Roper next says, "We know he wore no glasses: he is said to have waved them away the remark, 'Bon Dieu, je vois comme Bouguereau.'" I have tried, without success, to find another reference to this quotation of Renoir's seeing like Bouguereau, that is, seeing the world with too much detail.

A biography of Renoir warns us to be very careful in evaluating memoirs written long after the fact because they depend on distant memory: "After the artist's death, many of his friends and his son Jean wrote colorful, anecdotal accounts of his life and art."[11] Nevertheless, I feel that Jean Renoir's comments about his father's eyesight are important. He wrote that his father's vision remained keen up to his death and that "I can still see him applying a point of white, no larger than a pinhead, to his canvas to indicate a reflection in the eye of a model. . . . We had to use a magnifying glass to make out the details of the perfect likeness. He sometimes wore glasses for reading, but he did so chiefly to save his eyes. When he was in a hurry or whenever he mislaid his glasses, he managed quite well without them. Whenever the weather permitted, we liked to sit on the terrace in the evening and watch the fishermen at Cros-de-Cagnes sailing back to port. My father was always the first to spot a boat."[12]

The most reasonable conclusion is to discount the anecdotes about Renoir's alleged myopia and to accept Jean Renoir's account of his father's presbyopia. Renoir wore glasses occasionally, for reading. His distant vision was good. Many older individuals have good distant vision, particularly in bright sunlight, which illuminates the field and also makes the pupil small. A small pupil in the eye, like a small iris diaphragm in a camera, increases the depth of field and reduces the stray rays of light. The result is a clearer image. Renoir's form of Impressionism was a conscious stylistic choice, not an ocular aberration grafted on to a realistic method of depiction.

—— **REFERENCES** ——

1. Quoted in Gowing L: Renoir's sentiment and taste. *Renoir*, Abrams, New York, 1985, p. 35 (catalogue of 1985-1986 retrospective shown in London, Paris and Boston).
2. Quoted in White BE: *Renoir, His Life, Art, and Letters*, Abrams, New York, 1984, p.96 (letter by Renoir, dated February 13, 1880).
3. White,[2] p. 191.
4. Pissarro C: *Letters to His Son Lucien*, Santa Barbara, Calif., 1981, Peregrine Smith, p. 434 (edited by J Rewald).
5. White,[2] p. 213.
6. Renoir J: *Renoir My Father*, Little, Brown, Boston, 1962, pp. 32-33.
7. House J: *Renoir*, p. 278 (exhibition catalogue).
8. Ravin J: Geriatrics and painting, *Art Journal* 27:397, 1968.
9. Charman W, Evans N: Possible effects of changes in lens pigmentation on the colour balance of an artist's work, *Br J Physiol Optics* 31:23-31, 1976.
10. Trevor-Roper P: *The World through Blunted Sight*, Bobbs Merrill, New York, 1970, p. 33.
11. White,[2] p.7.
12. Renoir,[6] p. 264.

Chapter Four

EYE PROBLEMS ATTRIBUTED TO EL GRECO

James G. Ravin

When El Greco (1541-1614) burst on the scene in sixteenth-century Spain, his creations were unique and powerful. The conservatives were stunned when faced with a style so different from standard modes of representation. Some reactionaries responded by asking, rather snidely, if the artist's eyesight and mental state were defective. Although there is no evidence that his faculties were anything but normal, the same questions have persisted for centuries.

El Greco was the first great Spanish painter. His given name was Domenikos Theotokopoulos, but after leaving Greek territory the nickname he was given, El Greco (the Greek), stayed with him. He was born on the island of Crete, trained in Italy, and spent the last half of his life in Spain.

Little is known about his early years on Crete. Apparently his family was wealthy and socially prominent. He was trained in the Byzantine style of icon painting there, and the elongated figures typical of icons became an important feature of his mature style. At about age 27 El Greco moved to Venice, where he spent 3 years. Venice controlled Crete at that time, and the Italian city was the home of thousands of Greeks. Venice was then at the peak of its glory as the artistic center of Italy. Titian, Tintoretto, and Veronese all were painting actively, and El Greco learned from each of them. He must have found the Venetian use of bright colors, dramatic light, and movement appealing, for they became features of his own art.

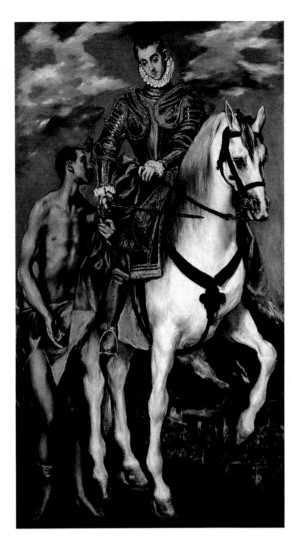

In 1570 he moved to Rome, where he saw the paintings of Raphael and Michelangelo. The nudes in Michelangelo's *Last Judgement* had offended some people, and repainting the figures was advised. El Greco is reported to have said that he could redo the painting "with honesty and decorum" and in "good quality." He also is quoted as saying that "Michelangelo was a good man, but he did not know how to paint."[1] El Greco did have great respect for Michelangelo as a draftsman. He also saw the paintings of Parmigianino, a virtuoso in the Mannerist style. His works are characterized by graceful, elongated figures and ambiguous space, features characteristic of El Greco's mature style.

When and why El Greco left Italy for Spain is not known. The plague of 1575 or the epidemic of the following year which killed Titian may have influenced him. In Rome he was at the center of intellectual circles, and he made contacts that most likely helped when he went to Spain. He certainly was aware that Spain was the most powerful country on earth and that its ruler, Philip II, sought artists to decorate his new palace and monastery, the Escorial. By 1577 he was in Spain. He apparently painted only one work for the king. After Philip rejected it, El Greco received no further royal commissions. But he was a popular artist. The church appreciated his humanistic and spiritualistic treatment of the Counter-Reformation themes. The many copies of his work done in the seventeenth century also attest to his popularity.

After he moved to Spain, El Greco's style matured. His unique style included elongated and isolated figures which exist in a strange type of space, nearly float-

ing (Fig. 4-1). This form of representation serves to emphasize the celestial quality of scenes that otherwise seem down to earth. The lighting is an eerie ghostlike
white, which evokes a strong emotional response in many viewers. This unique,
original style was controversial from its inception. El Greco did not satisfy King
Philip II, who preferred more conventional and mediocre artists, but he gained
much fame in Toledo. He was totally unconcerned with popular taste. He even
became involved in litigation about religious interpretations of his paintings and
the fees he had demanded

El Greco's art always has been popular in Spain, but he did not acquire an international reputation until the twentieth century. Interest was rekindled in the
1840s in France when his work was exhibited in the Louvre. Delacroix, Millet, and
Degas owned his paintings; Cézanne and Sargent copied him. Americans became
more aware of his work after the first book in English devoted to his art was published in the early twentieth century. Not every critic found his art appealing. One
author, writing in *Art News*, described his painting as a "jumble of carelessly
thrown together, badly drawn human figures not worth fifty dollars."[2] Today most
critics admire the dramatic lighting, brilliant colors, and movement of his figures.

ASTIGMATISM?

El Greco's style was so original that it shocked many observers. Some thought
he must have been mad, though all surviving records indicate he was perfectly
sane. Others suggested he had an ocular defect, astigmatism. El Greco is not the
only artist who has been called astigmatic. Holbein, Cranach the elder, Botticelli,
Titian, Modigliani, and Sargent also have been placed in this category.[3] Astigmatism
is an optical abnormality in which light rays from a single point are not focused at
a point on the retina but rather are spread out as a line in one direction.

There are two popular arguments in favor of the theory of astigmatism. First,
artists sometimes will distort objects in one direction. If an astigmatic lens is
placed over one eye of an artist and he is asked to draw a circle, he will draw an
ellipse. Second, if an astigmatic lens is used to view an El Greco painting, the
abnormal elongation of his figures can be made to disappear.

There are several arguments against the theory[4] however, and they may be
summarized as follows:

1. Elongation in El Greco's art is purely stylistic. He was influenced by the
   elongated figures of Byzantine art and the distortion of the Mannerist
   style of painting.
2. If an artist has astigmatism, elongation should occur in only one direction.
   But the distortion of El Greco's figures occurs in both the horizontal and
   vertical directions. Most of his bodies are stretched vertically yet have fingers stretched horizontally (Fig. 4-2). If astigmatism were the cause of vertical elongation, the horizontally placed fingers should have been portrayed as short and stubby.
3. Astigmatism usually does not change greatly over time. However, El
   Greco's distortions progressed markedly as he aged.
4. The celebrated painting *The Burial of the Count of Orgaz*, has normally pro-
   portioned figures in the lower part of the canvas and distorted ones in
   the upper regions of the same painting. An ocular abnormality cannot
   explain this.
5. Astigmatism should not affect an artist's works. If an artist attempts to
   paint realistically, the object and its painted image should correspond.
   Otherwise, when the artist compares the two, a discrepancy will be noted.

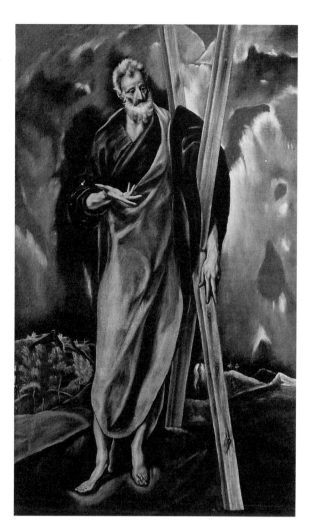

For example, if the artist sees in nature a point but paints it as an elongated line, when the artist looks at the painted line it will appear to be even more elongated. This logic seems compelling but in practice does not always work. Some astigmatic artists do distort along the line of their astigmatism.[3,5]

There is also one remote possibility. If El Greco had two dissimilar eyes, one farsighted and astigmatic and the other nearsighted, astigmatism could have had an effect. The farsighted eye could have been used for seeing the object to be painted and the nearsighted eye could have been used to view the canvas so that he would not be comparing the object and its painted image with the same eye. The arguments seem to favor the skeptics, but the answer awaits a prospective study of astigmatic artists.

CHANGES IN DETAILS AND COLOR

During El Greco's long artistic career, he often painted the same theme several times. There are, for example, several versions of *The Purification of the Temple* and *The Annunciation*. This gives us the opportunity to compare early and late works. Comparison of the purification canvases reveals a loss of details with time

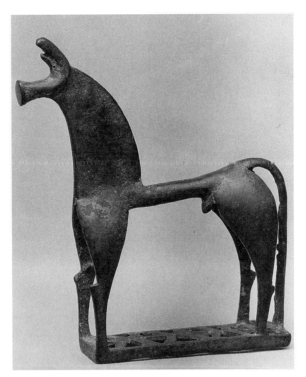

FIGURE 5 - 1

Bronze horse, third quarter of the
eighth century B.C. Height: 17.6
centimeters. *(All rights reserved, The
Metropolitan Museum of Art, New York,
Rogers Fund, 1921.)*

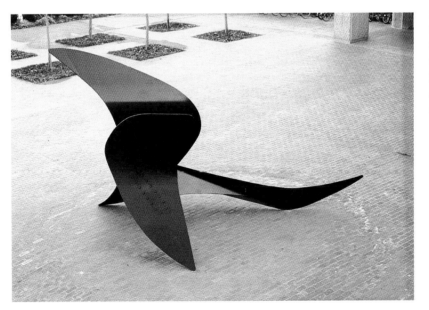

FIGURE 5 - 2

Calder. *Le Faucon (The Falcon).*
Painted steel, 1963 located in the
courtyard of the Stanford Law
School. *(Stanford University Museum of
Art [93.62]. Gift of Richard and June
Lang.)*

and confident in mastering ever more refined tools and techniques, grew increasingly eager to portray the world around them as accurately as they saw it.

By the end of the sixth century B.C., on the eve of the great world war with
Persia, sharp scrutiny and representation of reality prevailed in Greek art.
Nowhere is this more apparent than in the marble statues of men and women
dedicated to Athena on the Acropolis, statues that reveal both anatomical accu-
racy and, in their brooding facial features, the carvers' capacity to capture something of the emotional tenor of the times.[3] Not to be outdone by their contemporaries working in stone, the painters of red-figure vases seem to have been just
as interested in the precise depiction of the human body, in action and inaction,

FIGURE 5-3
Athenian black-figure oinochoe
(wine pourer) showing Herakles ver-
sus Antaios. c. 515 B.C. *(Stanford
University Museum of Art [61.69].
Museum Purchase Fund.)*

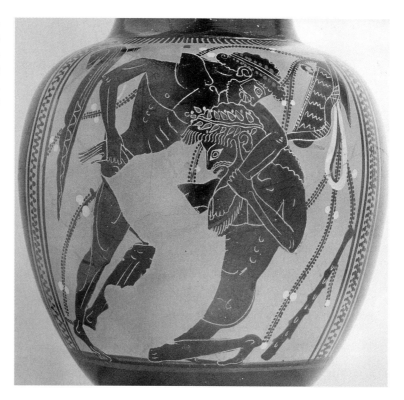

in all its complex beauty. They also conveyed, where appropriate, solemn and sometimes emotionally charged themes, in keeping with the somber mood of the day. Preeminent among these talented, ambitious painters was the Athenian master, Euphronios.[4] Born around the year 540 B.C., his career as a painter (c. 520-500) began soon after the invention of red-figure painting around 530 B.C. Prior to this, the favored technique had been black-figure: black silhouettes were painted on the orange surface of the vase, and details etched into the paint with a sharp tool and further enlivened with red and white color.[5] The charm as well as the limitations of this technique are evident in the wine pourer of around 530 B.C. with Herakles wrestling the Libyan giant, Antaios (Fig. 5-3).

Realizing that black-figure had been fully explored and exhausted by their elders, Euphronios' senior colleagues began to experiment with color reversal and soon came upon the more "painterly" and naturalistic possibilities of red-fig-ure: black outlines were painted around the contours of now "skin-colored" fig-ures, and internal details were applied with a black brush which, when diluted, produced an appealing honey color; then the background was blackened in. Once the new technique was mastered by the painters and embraced by their clientele, and once it was shown to be a trend with staying power, the craft could be taken to the next level by eager young men like Euphronios. He and his contemporaries began to explore the relatively rich opportunities offered by red-figure, such as modulations and subtleties of brush, that the less flexible etching tool of black-figure would not allow. These included raised relief lines for sharp contours, paler diluted lines to define rippling, subcutaneous musculature, and even the bold use of impasto—possibilities that the inventors of red-figure, preoccupied with the challenges of devising and popularizing the new technique, had not thought or sought to investigate.

In his depiction of Herakles wrestling the giant Antaios on a large mixing bowl (Fig. 5-4), Euphronios deployed his full arsenal of technical advantages, the bet-ter to bring out the contrast between the wily, civilized Herakles and his uncouth

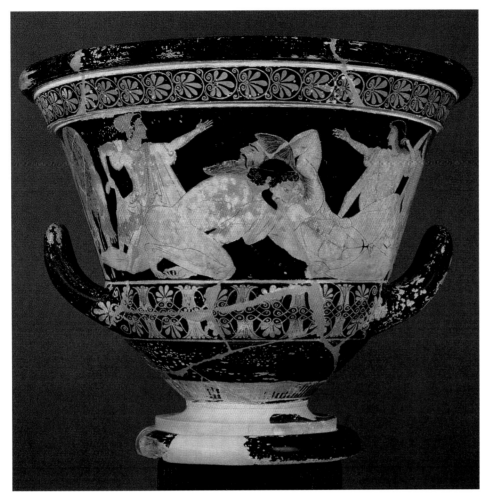

FIGURE 5-4

Euphronios. Athenian red-figure krater (mixing bowl) with Herakles versus Antaios. c. 520 B.C. *(Musée du Louvre, Paris. Copyright © Photo R.M.N.)*

Libyan opponent. Herakles has jet-black hair with rows of rich impasto curls that catch and reflect light, a carefully clipped beard and moustache framing a firmly set mouth, prominent eyelashes and an arched brow, all applied with a hand as sure as the hero's inevitable victory. His opponent, in contrast, though possessing an impressive set of rectus abdominis muscles (shaded with dilute paint to simulate the effect of flexion) and great upper body strength, also bears the characteristic attributes of a doomed barbarian. His stringy, matted hair and straggly beard are rendered with a scruffiness that only dry brush can evoke and that stands in stark contrast to the dapper Herakles.

The articulation of such contrasts, between Greek and non-Greek, was beyond the realm of black-figure (consider again Fig. 5-3 and the equally good looks of both Herakles and Antaios) and required of Euphronios a good deal of careful observation, imagination, and skill. Distinctions between Greek hero and alien adversary had first to be conjured up in his mind, then applied to bodies that appear to have been based on careful observation of real wrestlers[6] Good distance vision was required to see the contours of the bodies, and a steady, decisive hand to paint them. Fig. 5-5 shows a young man decorating a vase, which allows us to imagine how Euphronios might have looked at work.

Nowhere is his ability to integrate these powers of observation, imagination and manual dexterity more pronounced or subtle than on his famous (and later) mixing bowl in the Metropolitan Museum in New York (Fig. 5-6). The primary side of the krater captures a solemn, melancholy moment from the

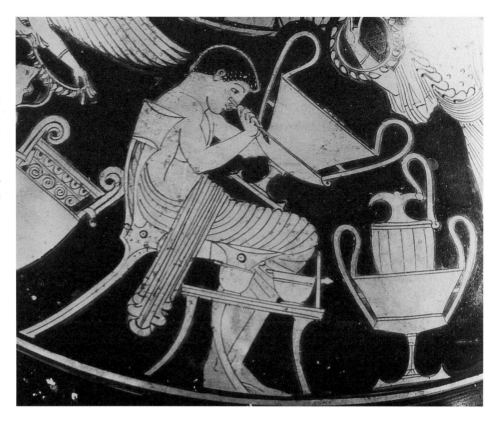

sixteenth book of Homer's *Iliad*: Sleep and Death, the winged twin brothers, bend down to lift the lifeless body of Zeus' son Sarpedon, fresh blood running in rivulets from puncture wounds to the thigh, abdomen and chest. Flanking the brothers are a pair of soldiers, sentinels with shield and spear, providing further closure to an already poignant study of life and death, age and youth, in elegiac opposition.

The artist's powers of observation—both at a distance and at extremely close range—are evident in the large, muscular bodies of the men, whose contours are as crisply defined as those of the bronze statues in Figs. 5-1 and 5-2. He may have studied models such as those who posed for contemporary grave stones, in which armed, stationary warriors carved in relief stand guard over their own tombs.[7] It is even possible to imagine Euphronios sketching the profiles of athletes in motion (such as Stanford cornerback Kwame Ellis, in Fig. 5-7) as preparatory studies for Sleep and Death. Having painted in the outlines for all the figures, he would then have pulled his chair close to the workbench, assembled his finest brushes and set to work on the exquisite details which make the figures, living and dead, so poignantly real. The greatest concentration of such details occurs on the figure of Death whose eyelashes, tiny dotted scales on wings and corslet and finely pleated undergarment draw our eye to his side of the picture, where even more minutely painted lashes, teeth and wavy hair are found on Sarpedon. Fingernails and toenails, ulnae and malleoli of corpse and caretakers, as well as the creases along Sarpedon's right index finger, would have required the finest of brushes and the sharpest of eyes held, like the nose of young Updike, a mere inch from the vase.

One of the mysterious aspects of the career of this "elite" artist is his abrupt abandonment of the profession of painting. After he finished the Sarpedon krater, which is dated around 510 B.C.,[8] he continued for another decade to paint vases and drinking cups made for him by collaborating potters. Then, around 500 B.C.,

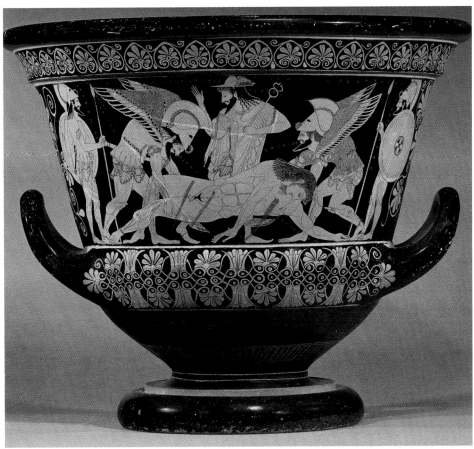

FIGURE   5-6

Euphronios. Athenian red-figure krater with Sleep and Death lifting the body of Sarpedon, c. 515 B.C. Also signed by Euxitheos as potter. Detail below of Thanatos (Death): note the fine brushwork and details. *(The Metropolitan Museum of Art, New York, Purchase, Bequest of Joseph H. Durkee, Gift of Darius Ogden Mills and Gift of C Ruxton Love, by exchange, 1972 Copyright © 1972 by The Metropolitan Museum of Art. All rights reserved.)*

Detail Figure 5-6

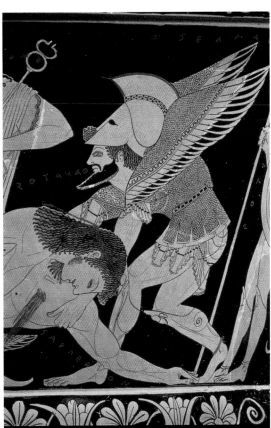

FIGURE 5-7

Stanford defensive back Kwame Ellis
in a stance similar to the one used by
Euphronios in his krater. (Peninsula
Times Tribune, *autumn 1992.
Photograph by Tim Berger.)*

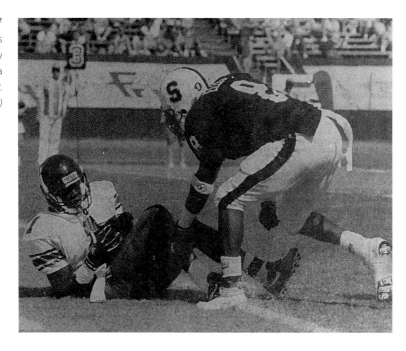

he put down his brush forever. None of his latest vases is as ambitious or dazzling as the Sarpedon krater though none gives evidence of a wavering hand or burnt-out soul. Did he leave his workshop to join his fellow Athenians in the campaigns (beginning in 499 B.C.) leading up to the Persian invasion of Marathon in 490 B.C., or did he die? These possibilities are ruled out by evidence of his persistent presence in Athens, for the duration of the Persian Wars and beyond, as a *potter* for other red-figure painters. His signature followed by the verb *epoiesen* (generally thought to mean "potted," though some have argued that the word denotes ownership of the workshop)[9] appears throughout the war years (499-479 B.C.) on vases decorated and signed by other painters. He lived long enough (at least beyond the age of 60) to serve as a potter for the Pistoxenos Painter. A cup in Berlin, dated to 470 B.C. and attributed to the Pistoxenos Painter, bears the latest extant signature "Euphronios *epoiesen.*"[10]

What would have prompted such a vocational shift, from consummate painter to either potter or entrepreneur? Sir John Beazley considered the possibility of bad eyesight, among other possibilities, as early as 1944: "We cannot know what led Euphronios to turn from decorating vases to shaping them. A mishap; change in eyesight—there were no spectacles to correct such changes—; the legitimate desire for a still better living. He may actually have preferred shaping vases to decorating them."[11] Remembering that Euphronios was born around 540 B.C. and that he would have been approximately 40 years old when he quit painting, the problem may simply have been presbyopia. A small child can practically see the tip of the nose, but between ages 45 and 50 an adult who sees clearly at a distance (either naturally or wearing spectacles) will begin to have trouble with reading and other close work (see Chapters 1 and 2). A myopic individual may not need reading glasses, of course, but at the price of poor vision (without glasses) at a distance. However, a hyperopic (farsighted) individual will start having difficulty with near work at an even younger age. Euphronios may have been mildly hyperopic.

It is perhaps puzzling, given the intellectual sophistication and technical ingenuity of the ancient Greeks, that no optical aids for presbyopia were available. It is even unclear to what extent the Greeks recognized presbyopia as a medical ail-

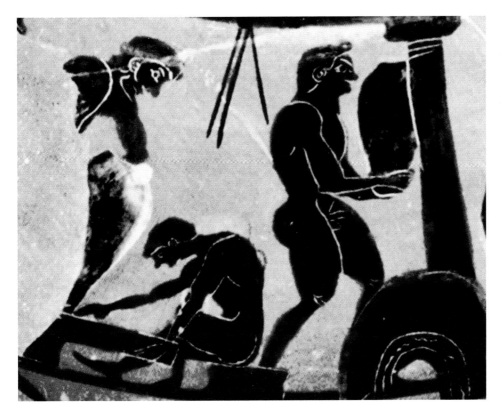

FIGURE 5-8

Artist from the Leagros Group. Detail of an Athenian black-figure hydria showing a potter at work, 520 B.C. *(Staatliche Antikensammlungen [Foto Museum], Munich.)*

ment, since it is not mentioned in the extant medical texts. The phenomenon was known, of course; Oribasius (a Greek physician from the third century A.D.) wrote that "the vision of old people is opposite to that of myopes: the first do not see clearly what is close, but see well at a distance."[12] However, the cure he recommended was far from optical and far from likely to help: a fortifying ointment of pomegranate juice and honey for printmakers, painters, and goldsmiths.[13] The ancient Greek language had no word specifically to describe the disorder. *Presbys* and *presbytes* refer to an old man, an elder, an ambassador, but *presbyopia* appears to be a modern word, coined within the past few centuries out of analogy with myopia and related terms.

Julius Hirschberg states definitively in the first volume of his 11-volume *History of Ophthalmology* that "spectacles were completely unknown in ancient Greece and Rome,"[13] although it was recognized that a hollow glass sphere filled with water could magnify objects. Seneca (4 B.C.-A.D. 65), the Roman philosopher and tutor of Nero, observed that "letters, however tiny and obscure, are seen larger and clearer when viewed through a glass ball filled with water."[14] Such spheres may have been used sporadically by elderly Greeks, but no description of their regular use as a cure or device for presbyopia has been discovered. The Greek scholar John Boardman was also convinced that Greek artisans did their fine work with the naked eye. In his discussion of ancient Greek makers of gems and finger rings, Boardman notes that "although the magnifying effect of crystal or glass in lens form may well have been observed at an early date, it is highly improbable that it was exploited by artists. No deliberately fashioned lenses have been found and it is unlikely that Pliny would have failed to mention their use."[15]

If Euphronios was presbyopic, and intended to remain actively engaged in his chosen profession, he would have been forced to modify his activity to avoid close work. As a potter for other painters, he could have functioned effectively without having to depend on extreme proximity to the clay, as required for the meticulous painting of vases and cups. This is illustrated in both the black-figure potter in Fig. 5-8 and in the photograph of Georgia O'Keeffe (see Fig. 19-7). In each instance, the detached gaze and distance of potter from pot are different from the intense close scrutiny of the painter that was evident in Fig. 5-5. The shaping of vases on a potter's wheel would have allowed Euphronios to work at a greater distance from the clay, since the building of walls and refining of contours depend more on subtlety of palm and fingertips than on coordination of brush, hand, and eye. Indeed, it was for these reasons that artists such as Degas (see Chapter 17) and O'Keeffe (see Chapter 19) turned to sculpture and potting when their vision failed. And if *epoiesen* should have meant that he owned and operated the workshop, the inability to "focus inside of two feet" never impeded anyone from supervising and deriving financial profit from the sweat and toil of others. Either as potter or businessman, he could have continued his ceramic career as a presbyope.

It may be relevant that Euphronios dedicated an offering to Athena on the Athenian Acropolis some 20 years later (just after 480 B.C.).[16] An inscribed pillar monument there bears the name of Euphronios as *kerameus* (potter) and specifies the recipient as Athena *hygieia*. This designation is important for it identifies Athena in her capacity as overseer of health and healing, one of her many responsibilities in the sixth and fifth centuries B.C., well before the establishment of 420 B.C. of a sanctuary of Asklepios on the south slope of Acropolis. The inscription almost certainly identifies the red-figure-painter-turned-potter (not some hitherto unknown potter of the same name) appealing to Athena for a cure of an unspecified malady or mishap. Whether his supplication to her was prompted by ophthalmological problems, such as presbyopia, glaucoma, or cataracts, or by some other disorder, we cannot determine. It may be significant that some 40% of the votive body parts placed by later pilgrims in the shrine of Asklepios are models of eyes.[17] It may be that Asklepios' fame as an eye specialist was inherited from his predecessor, Athena, whose ophthalmological fame extends as far back as the Trojan War (twelfth century B.C.), in which Homer describes her having removed mist from the eyes of Diomedes. With respect to Euphronios, we cannot know for sure whether deteriorating eyesight or some other concern prompted his appeal to Athena, nor can we tell if Athena answered it with a cure or patiently presided over time's capacity to heal. We do know that he could continue to work as a potter, as suggested by his potter signature on the aforementioned drinking cup decorated by the Pistoxenos Painter around 470 B.C.

Euphronios did not have the good fortune to spend his entire career painting, but other Greek vase painters enjoyed long careers. The Amasis Painter, the old black-figure impresario, maintained his keen eye and jeweller's touch, decorating large and small vases alike, from about 560 until 515 B.C. (when he would have been at least 60 years old) Dietrich von Bothmer speculated as a result that he was myopic and thus able to see well at close range even in his older years.[18] Perhaps it was nearsightedness that had spurred the young Amasis Painter to concentrate on decorating vases rather than on art forms more dependent on distant observation. Or perhaps his myopia was in part a result of years of intense close work during his youth and apprenticeship (see Fig. 5-5). There is evidence that extensive near work and reading may be one factor contributing to the development of myopia in modern society—a problem that physicians are hoping to resolve. In ancient Greece, paradoxically, the disease may also have been the cure for long-lived vase painters and others whose livelihood depended on detailed close work.

Euphronios serves as a reminder that many ancient people whose work obliged them to operate at close range—jewellers, coin makers, gem cutters, vase painters, dentists, and scribes—would at middle age have faced the progressive blurring of objects that they had been accustomed to seeing clearly. Unless they were tenacious and resourceful enough to find new employment that did not require the sharp near acuity of their younger years, such persons and their families would have suffered, even starved. Homer, himself blind, was a paragon of such adaptability, and when he called his hero Odysseus *polytropos*—an epithet implying versatile, ingenious, crafty, turning in many ways—he could as well have been describing Euphronios, painter, potter, and presbyope.

REFERENCES

1. Updike J: *Collected Poems, 1953-1993*, Alfred A. Knopf, New York, 1995, p. 356. Copyright © 1993 by John Updike. Reprinted by permission of Alfred A. Knopf, Inc. and Penguin Books Ltd.

2. Paton WR (trans): *The Greek Anthology*, William Heinemann, London, 1925 (Book IX: epigrams 734 and 731, translated anew. Epigrams 713-742 and 793-798 all concern Myron's cow).

3. See some of the late-sixth- and early-fifth-century images of men and women in Richter GMA: *Kouroi*, Phaidon, London, 1970, figs. 564-571; *Korai*, Phaidon, London, 1968, figs. 411-419; Payne HGG, Young GM, *Archaic Marble Sculpture from the Athenian Acropolis*, William Morrow, New York, 1950, plates 70-71, 75-78, 83-88, 109-115.

4. The most recent publications on the painter were generated by a traveling exhibition of his work and a series of colloquia. Illustrated catalogues: *Capolavori de Euphronios*, Fabbri, Milan, 1990; *Euphronios: Pittore ad Atene nel VI secolo a. C.*, Fabbri, Milan, 1991; *Euphronios der Maler*, Fabbri, Milan, 1991. Colloquia: Cygielman M et al (eds): *Euphronios: Atti del seminario internazionale distudi*, Il Ponte, Florence, 1992; Denoyelle M (ed): *Euphronios peintre*, Documentation Francaise, Paris, 1992; Wehgartner I (ed): *Euphronios und seine Zeit* (Staatliche Museen zu Berlin: Preussischer Kulturbesitz, Berlin, 1992).

5. The standard work on techniques of painting and potting is Nobel JV: *The Techniques of Painted Attic Pottery*, rev ed, Thames and Hudson, London, 1988.

6. For a splendid modern reenactment of this pose and an important study of Euphronios' anatomical drawing, see Kurtz DC: Pioneering anatomical realism, in Cygielman M et al (eds),[4] pp. 29-35, plates XXXIII-XLIX, with the wrestlers on plate XXXVII. Mr. Robert Hatta, a Stanford student-wrestler, notes that Herakles engages in what is still today recognized in collegiate, Greco-Roman, and freestyle/international competitions as the "pull-back" or "suck-back."

7. Compare with Richter GMA: *The Archaic Gravestones of Attica*, Phaidon, London, 1961, figs. 129 and 156-158.

8. For the relative chronology of his work, see Dietrich von Bothmer's chart in the catalogue *Euphronios: pittore ad Atene nel VI secolo a.C.* (Fabbri, Milan, 1991) p. 268.

9. On the various meanings of *epoiesen* see Cook RM: *Epoiesen* on Greek vases, *JHS* 91:137-138, 1971; Robertson M: *Epoiesen* on Greek vases: Other considerations, *JHS* 92:180-183, 1972; Eisman M: A further note on *epoiesen* signatures, *JHS* 94:172, 1974.

10. Berlin F2282: Antikenmuseum Staatliche Museen Preussischer Kulturbesitz: *ARV*, 859 no. 1; *Beazley Addenda*, 2, p. 298; illustrated in the catalogue *Euphronios pittore ad Atene nel VI secolo a.C.* (Fabbri, Milan, 1991) pp. 226-229.

11. Beazley JD: Potter and painter in ancient Athens. In DC Kurtz (ed): *Greek Vases: Lectures by JD Beazley*, Clarendon Press, Oxford, 1989, pp. 39-59. Quote is from p. 55.

12. Quoted in Hirschberg J: *The History of Ophthalmology*, Wayenborgh, Bonn, 1982 (translated by FC Blodi, vol. I, p. 108).

13. Hirschberg,[12] p. 159.

14. Seneca, *Naturales quaestiones* I, 6.5, Harvard University Press, Cambridge, 1971 (translated by TH Corcoran).

15. Boardman J: *Greek Gems and Finger Rings*, Abrams, New York, 1972, p. 382.

16. Discussed by Maxmin J: Euphronios *epoiesen*: Portrait of the artist as a presbyopic potter. In ACF Verity, P Walcot (eds): *Greece & Rome*, vol. 21 Clarendon Press, Oxford, 1974, pp. 178-180. For the definitive description of the pillar monument, see Raubitschek AE: *Dedications from the Athenian Acropolis* Archaeological Institute of America, Cambridge, Mass., 1949, pp. 211-258, with archaeological and epigraphic references on p. 255.

17. See Maxmin,[16] p. 180. Euphronios' supplication to Athena, like so much else in ancient Greek culture, finds contemporary parallels in the silver icons of bodies, body parts, internal organs, babies, animals, houses, cars, motorcycles, and so on dedicated in modern Greek churches.

18. von Bothmer D: *The Amasis Painter and His World*, J. Paul Getty Museum, Malibu, Calif., 1985, p.43.

Part Three

LIGHT VERSUS DARK

Chapter Six

THE BANDS OF ERNST MACH

EDGE EFFECTS IN ART

Michael F. Marmor

Czech scientist Ernst Mach (1838-1916) was a Renaissance man. Physicist, psychologist, and philosopher, he made contributions in a variety of disciplines that influenced the course of modern scientific thinking.[1,2] He championed "positivism" in science, which demanded vigorous experimental proof for concepts and theories, even those as broad as "time" and "space." In fact, the problems that physicists encountered in trying to define time and space so rigorously laid a foundation for the development of the theory of relativity by Einstein.

Early in his career, Mach was intrigued by perception, and he studied the curious bands of lightness or darkness that appeared on shadows and at the borders of regions that differed in brightness. These phenomena (now called Mach bands) were not new; they had been observed by other psychologists and used by artists for millenia. However, Mach had the insight to recognize that the enhancements of contrast at borders might derive from physiologic processes within the retina and were not simply matters of psychological interpretation. He was ahead of his time, since the anatomic and physiologic evidence for inhibitory and excitatory neural convergence within the retina (see Chapter 1) would not appear for the better part of a century. Mach's name may be known best now for his definition of air speed as a function of the local speed of sound. However, while Mach 1 may be faster than most of us will travel, Mach bands appear in many aspects of our daily life and are an important feature of both the production and appreciation of art.

An illustration of Mach bands, as they may appear at the edge of sharply cast shadows, appears in Fig. 6-1, Mach bands are present wherever gradations of brightness meet at a sharp boundary. They reflect neural connections in the retina and brain that makes us more sensitive to differences in brightness than to steady light or dark itself (see Chapter 1). These cues at borders are so powerful in guiding our perception that the presence of a Mach band can *create* a sense of lightness or darkness on either side that doesn't actually exist (Fig. 6-2). Other examples of Mach bands are illustrated in Chapter 1 (see Figs. 1-7 and 1-8).

Both perceived Mach bands (i.e., narrow bands of light or dark that are seen at a border as in Fig. 6-1) and illusory phenomena produced as a result of Mach bands (as in Fig. 6-2) have been used—at times intentionally and at times unconsciously—throughout the history of art. Some of the first examples of Mach bands appear in wall paintings from Pompeii and Herculaneum, created between the second century B.C. and the time of Vesuvius' eruption in A.D. 79. Some of this art is based on earlier Greek styles, the originals of which have been lost, so the use of Mach bands in Western art may extend back even further than Pompeii. The Roman painters used Mach bands in several different ways, and they appear to have been quite aware of the visual phenomenon. Fig. 6-3 shows a detail from a still life in which overlapping shadows behind the birds show crisp Mach bands. Mach effects also appear in the architectural perspective paintings which adorn some of the villa walls, to enhance the sense of depth and the trompe l'oeil effect of painted columns and porticos.

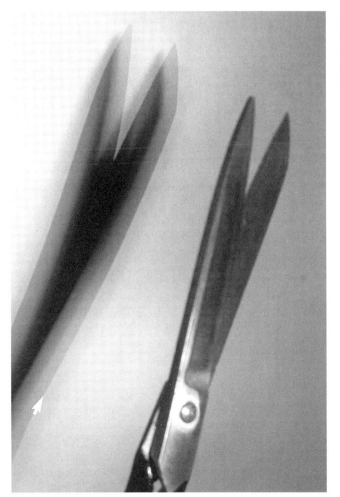

FIGURE 6-1
Shadows of scissor blades showing Mach bands at junctions of different density. Note the apparent white line that rings the darker shadow *(arrow)*.

FIGURE   6-2

Illusion of darkness and lightness produced by the presence of Mach bands. The central region appears darker because of Mach bands on either side. Masking the junctions (e.g., by holding up pencils) will show that all three regions are the same *(After an illusion shown by Burr.[7])*

Mach band effects are an important component of ancient and traditional Asian painting, particularly brush painting in which lightness and darkness are portrayed by shading rather than solid colors. Fig. 6-4 shows a striking example in which strong Mach bands make the mountains appear dark, although in fact only the borders are darker than the surrounding sky; conversely, the dark band about the moon makes it appear as a bright object in the sky, although its core is little brighter than the surrounding sky. The use of these effects can be traced back to at least the T'ang Dynasty in China (A.D. 618-907). They may have been used even earlier, but original art works were not preserved. A copy of the great scroll by Gu Kaizhi (Ku K'ai-chih, c. A.D. 345-406) shows subtle shading and some Mach band effects, but the copy was done hundreds of years later and we do not know whether the same pattern of shading was in the original. By the tenth and eleventh centuries, Chinese artists had become quite accomplished in the use of Mach bands. It is interesting that whereas the Greek and Roman artists mostly portrayed perceptual bands, the Asian artists created Mach band effects in order to generate illusions of lightness or darkness in space. They may have lacked Mach's insight into retinal circuitry, but they clearly recognized the illusory power of contrast.

Mach bands largely disappeared from Western art during the Dark Ages when perspective and shadows were abandoned in favor of iconography. But they reappeared in the Renaissance. As in Greek and Roman art, their use was generally the depiction of bands at the edges of objects and shadows. They reflected the artists' recognition of these perceptual phenomena more than a technique to create illusory effects. Some remarkable examples appear in the precise paintings of the Dutch master of Flémalle, Robert Campin, who was active from 1406 to 1444 (Fig. 6-5). He was obviously fascinated by shadows and painted them with exquisite precision, often showing double or triple shadows as may occur from multiple sources of light. Note the similarity between the shadow effects in Fig. 6-5 and those in Fig. 6-3. In some of the shadows, there is a clear dark band at the edge, and a light band adjacent, indicating that Campin not only recognized the perception of Mach bands but was trying to duplicate them in his art. The painted bands are more extreme than one usually observes in nature, but the

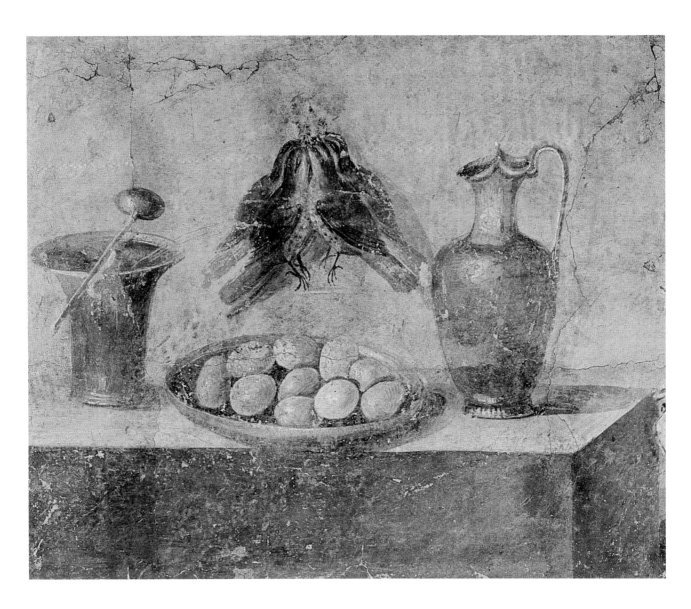

artist was clearly trying to put in the picture what he saw—perhaps not realizing that perceptual Mach bands would automatically appear as long as he painted shadows with a sharp edge.

The Italian painter Montegna (1431-1506) drew Mach bands into some of his pictures, and Leonardo da Vinci (1452-1519) described Mach bands very clearly in his writings: "The border of a vertical rod will appear very dark against a white field, and against a dark background it will appear brighter than any part of the rod, even though the light striking the latter is equally bright all along."[3] Some of his drawings show experimentation with heightened border contrast (Fig. 6-6), a technique we have already seen in Fig. 6-5.

The lightening or darkening of borders to enhance contrast is a device used consciously by many painters since Leonardo's time. The neo-Impressionists were particularly fascinated by this phenomenon, and Mach bands are unusually prominent in the works of Seurat, Signac, and others of this school.[4] Note in the sketch of a seated boy (Fig. 6-7) how the wall lightens behind his back and right calf, but darkens in front of his arm and leg. The wall becomes a somewhat irrational mixture of light and dark that bears no relationship to illumination or shadows. Here Mach bands have run amok and threatened to interfere with,

FIGURE   6-3

Anonymous. *Still Life with Eggs and Birds.*

Detail of roman wall painting.

(Scala/Art Resource, NY. Museo Archeologico Nazionale, Naples, Italy.)

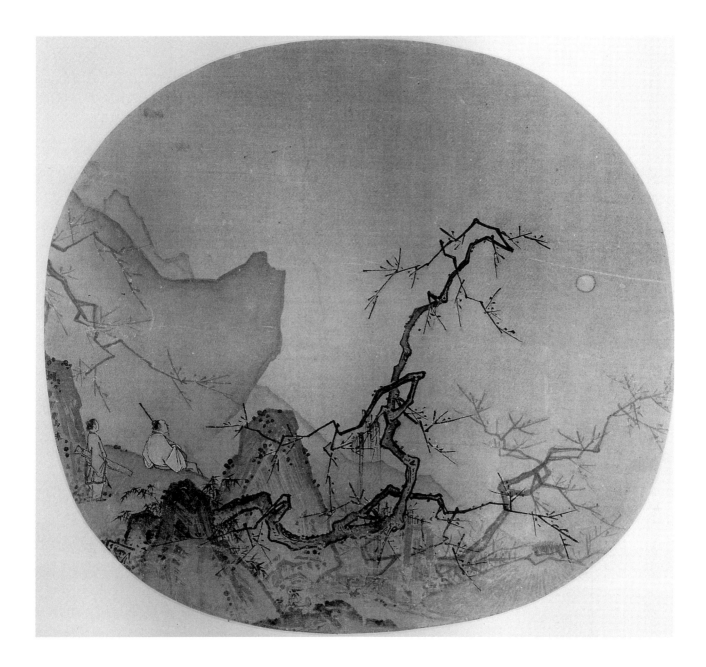

rather than enhance, the picture. This extreme use of border contrast by Seurat is not an accident, however, and he used similar effects in many of his drawings and in well-known oils such as *The Bathers* (for which Fig. 6-7 is a study) and *Les Poseuses* (for which Figs. 11-5 and 11-10 are studies). In part, he was trying to follow the dictates of scientists and art theorists who emphasized the importance of contrast in making objects distinct and luminous. This principle can be traced back to Leonardo's writings, and while we have no record that Seurat read Leonardo, we know that he studied carefully Sutter's *Les Phénomènes de la Vision* and Blanc's *Grammaire des Arts du Dessin*, which echoed Leonardo's ideas. Blanc wrote: "Leonardo da Vinci says we should place a light background in contrast to a shadow and a dark background to a mass of light, and it is a general principle, a precept not to be attacked."[5]

A number of twentieth-century artists have used Mach bands to augment their vision of the world. Two notable examples are Georgia O'Keeffe (see Fig. 6-8) and

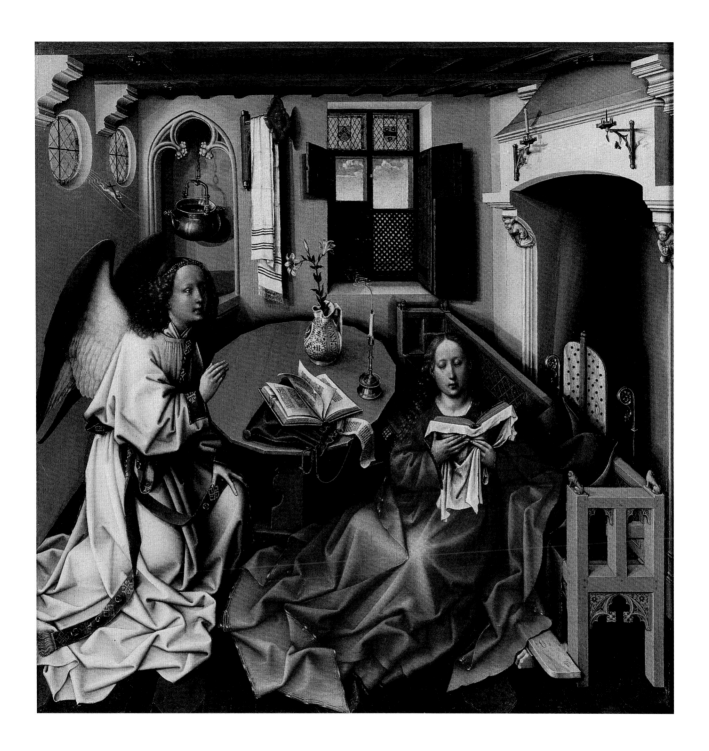

Arthur Dove (Fig. 6-9). These two American artists have much in common, for they shared an ability to see abstract forms in nature and to focus attention on the colors and shapes of a scene independent of its figurative content. Both worked in the first half of the twentieth century, and they shared the patronage and friendship of Alfred Stieglitz. Dove maintained this relationship with Stieglitz until 1946 when both men died; O'Keeffe married Stieglitz, of course, and continued to paint for another 30 years after his death. Stieglitz was one of the few dealers to recognize Dove's talent early in the century, and his patronage literally kept Dove alive during the depression (along with purchases and gifts from the

FIGURE 6-5

Campin. *The Annunciation.*

Oil on wood.

(The Metropolitan Museum of Art. Copyright © 1956 by The Metropolitan Museum of Art. All rights reserved. The Cloisters Collection, 1956.)

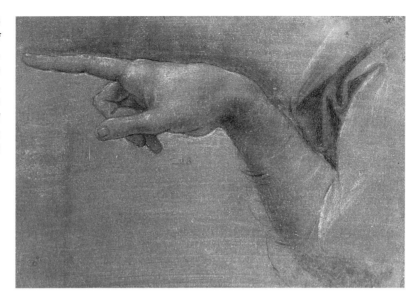

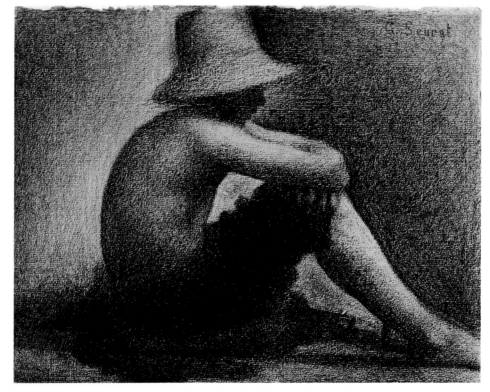

Washington collector, Duncan Phillips). Although one can find similarity in the artistic approaches of O'Keeffe and Dove, it is interesting that they used Mach bands in different ways. O'Keeffe produced Mach effects at borders to enhance the lightness or darkness of space, such as in the walls of the Taos church and in banks of clouds or mountains (see Fig. 19-1), much in the fashion of Asian brush painters. However, Dove painted adjacent or concentric bands of color that increased gradually in density and created strong Mach band perceptions. He called these gradations "power bands" and was fascinated by their effect, although I know of no evidence that he had ever analyzed them from a physiologic vantage point.

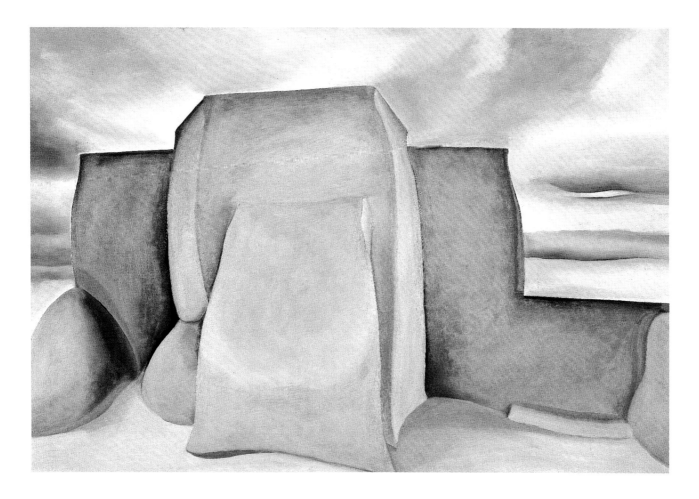

FIGURE 6-8
O'Keeffe. *Ranchos Church-Taos.*
Oil on canvas, 1930. *(Amon Carter Museum, Fort Worth, Texas, 1971.16)*

Modern optical artists, not surprisingly, have also been fascinated by the visual effects of Mach bands. These bands have been used strikingly by Vasarely (Fig. 6-10) to produce figures rife with bands generated by a progression of graded color densities. One can argue, of course, whether these effects represent art or simply decoration and whether the Mach bands in Dove's or Vasarely's paintings are artistic genius or merely visual games with a psychology experiment. I would argue that our physiologic understanding of Mach band illusions is quite irrelevant to whether an artist uses them in art. No one would say that the recent cloning of the genes for retinal color pigments[6] diminishes in any way the fact that Monet painted in color. Dove, Vasarely, and also Montegna, Campin, and countless Asian brush painters have either painted or generated Mach bands because they are a component of normal visual experience, just like color, shadow, texture, and movement. The measure of a painting is whether the visual tools have been used effectively to challenge and engage the viewer, not which technique has been used. Recognizing how Mach bands are a component of a work of art neither denigrates nor elevates the status of that art; it simply allows the viewer to appreciate better what the artist perceived or was trying to achieve.

It should also be noted that some artists have achieved their artistic goals by avoiding or obliterating Mach bands and border contrast. One of the striking characteristics of Renoir's work is the "softness" of his female faces and figures, rather like the misty cinematography of the heroine in an old movie. How did Renoir achieve this? Careful inspection of his canvases (Fig. 6-11) shows that he diffuses the sharp border around faces or nude figures with a relatively broad line of paint that has a density or color intermediate between that of the flesh and the

FIGURE 6-9
Dove. *Fog Horns.*
Oil, 1929. *(Colorado Springs
Fine Arts Center.)*

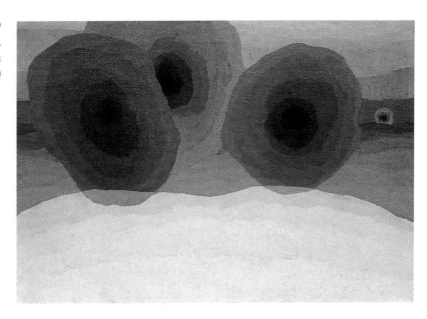

FIGURE 6-10
Vasarely. *Torony III.*
Lithograph, 1988 *(© 1996 Artists
Rights Society [ARS], New York/ADAGP,
Paris. Private Collection.)*

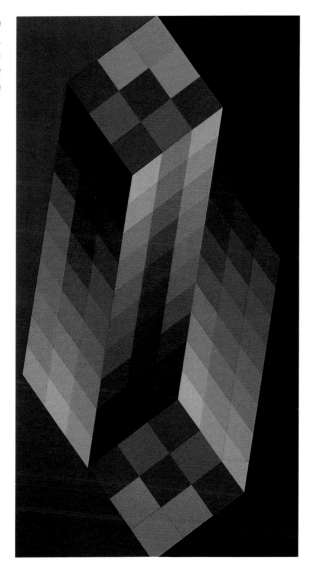

Detail Figure 6-11

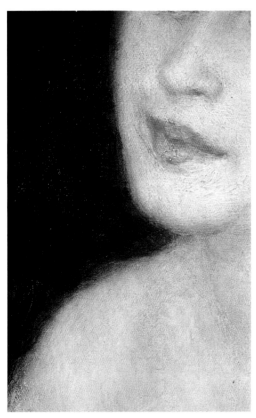

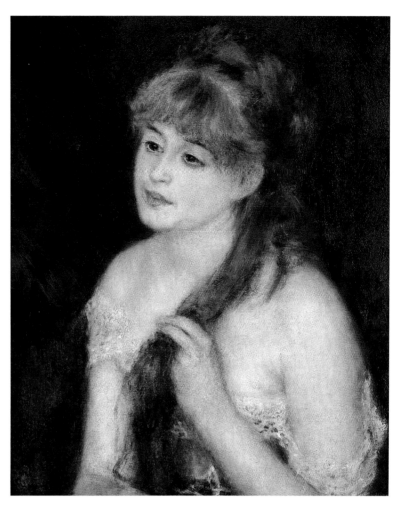

surrounding background. In other words, he did the opposite of what Leonardo recommended and he created a graded intermediate zone between the skin and its surround, thereby eliminating Mach bands, diminishing the sense of contrast, and blurring the sense of form. This technique contributes to the "softness" of figures in the work of other painters as well, such as Correggio.

Ernst Mach did not invent the phenomenon of Mach bands, since they reside within us all, and he was not the first to observe them, since artists have depicted them for two millenia. However, he had the insight to recognize that they derive from the eye itself, from the excitatory and inhibitory signals that craft our sensitivity to contrast. The phenomenon may have been used by artists for many centuries, but it is the legacy of Mach that we can understand why.

FIGURE   **6-11**

Renoir. *Young Woman Braiding Her Hair.*

Oil, 1876. Note the thick border of intermediate and graded tonality along the woman's right cheek, shoulder, and arm (detail at left). This diminishes the contrast between her skin and the background, and creates a soft and almost indeterminate border to her body. *(Ailsa Mellon Bruce Collection, © 1996 Board of Trustees, National Gallery of Art, Washington, D.C.)*

— REFERENCES —

1. Ratliff F: *Mach Bands: Quantitative Studies on Neural Networks in the Retina*, Holden-Day, San Francisco, 1965.
2. Cohen RS, Seeger RJ (eds): *Ernst Mach. Physicist and Philosopher*, D. Reidel, Dordrecht, 1970.
3. Weale RA: Discoverer of Mach-bands, *Invest Ophthalmol Vis Sci* 18:652-654, 1979.
4. Ratliff FA: *Paul Signac and Color in Neo-Impressionism*, Rockefeller University Press, New York, 1992.
5. Homer WI: *Seurat and the Science of Painting*, MIT Press, Cambridge, Mass., 1964, pp. 85-86.
6. Nathans J, Thomas D, Hogness DS: Molecular genetics of human color vision: The genes encoding blue, green, and red pigments, *Science* 232:193-232, 1986.
7. Burr DC: Implications of the Craik-O'Brien illusion for brightness perception, *Vision Res* 27:1903-1913, 1987.

Chapter Seven

A MATTER OF ILLUMINATION

Robert A. Weale

THE PROBLEM

Until 20 or 25 years ago, there used to hang in the foyer of the National Gallery in London a remarkable painting by the seventeenth-century Dutch artist Gerrit van Honthorst (Fig. 7-1). It represents Christ before the high priest, the former standing, as befits a defendant, and the latter seated, as is appropriate to one legally superior to the other. They are painted against murky background, at the back of which one can discern some nosy onlookers. But the center of the scene is occupied by a flame. It burns brightly and coincides with the point of intersection of the diagonals of the picture: we face a monument to a candle.

Hanging where it used to, and illuminated by bluish north daylight through the ceiling, the painting appeared to be submerged in an unreal pink aura. This suggests that that light differed from the illumination prevalent during its production. And that is, in fact, the case. The artist, who spent many years in Rome, was known there as Gherardo delle notte (Gerard of the nights) because he frequently painted in the dark by torch light. This explains why *Christ before the High Priest* appears pink in ordinary daylight. In the mid-1970s, the painting was cleaned and moved into an area where it is now lit by warm incandescent light, the tonality of which more nearly approaches that of the light of a torch: lo and behold! the pink has vanished, and the impression of the painting has been "right" ever since.

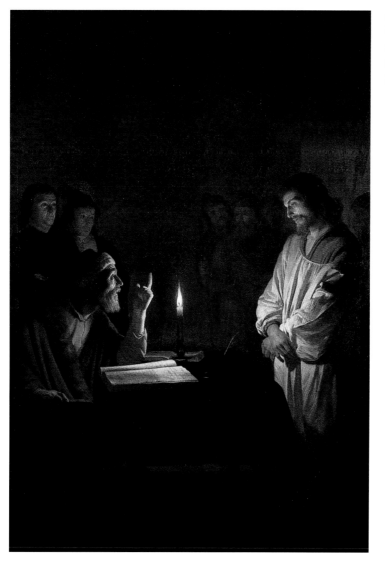

There are those who argue that the painting of, and in, artificial light offers no problem to overcome. The rationale of this view is that the artist knows how to compensate for differences in lighting in general, particularly when the location a painting is destined for is known. It has even been suggested that paintings apparently created in artificial light were, in fact, painted by daylight.

There is categorical evidence to oppose this. Rembrandt's pupil Gerard Dou produced a panel presenting a painter painting by candlelight. The single candle shown testifies more to the painter's poverty than his good sense, but the message is clear: it documents the use of artificial light for the purpose of painting. Over 100 years later, Goya painted a self-portrait which is now in the Prado in Madrid. He is wearing a hat, and around its brim there are a number of lit candles, the object of which is unmistakable: they served to light the canvas while he was painting.

The moral of this is lost on many directors of picture galleries who continue to believe that illuminating their treasures by daylight is the acme of perfection. It is therefore interesting to try to trace how artists tackled a variety of lighting situations through the ages and to determine how we should respond to their endeavors.

LIGHT IS GOD

There are two ways in which an artist can indicate what type of illumination strikes the scene he is depicting. One is the information conveyed by shadows, the other by color. To take color first, consider the difference between sunlight and moonlight. The former is warm, the latter cool. The former will emphasize the red and orange end of the spectrum, the latter more nearly the green and blue side. We shall see later that a skilled artist like Piero della Francesca had mastered the characteristics of different types of light so well as to be able to utilize them in conveying assorted atmospheres and moods.

Historically speaking, the matter of shadows is more interesting. The reason is that they were not used in certain periods. The Romans used them in Pompeii, and they can be seen also in the large mosaics in the Bardo Museum in Tunis. But in medieval paintings shadows are obtrusive by their absence, only to reappear very tentatively toward the end of the fifteenth century.

As they must have been visible even in medieval days, one asks why they were not painted. The reason turns out to be theological. Many are the times when the Divine Light was seen as a literal entity: God was light. But the omnipresence of the Deity implied that there could not be any part of the universe where light failed to reach. In particular, God was deemed to be everywhere at the then center of the universe, namely the earth. But if an artist had painted a shadow, he would have pointed at an absence of light, and therefore be held to question divine omnipresence. That candle was not worth the game, and shadows were therefore ignored.

This explains why the so-called primitives, for a fourteenth-century example, relied on outlining their people and objects in terms of color. The same is true of Matisse in the twentieth century. Admittedly, the latter did so under the influence of Eastern art: no shadow appears in Japanese woodcuts, in Chinese paintings on silk, or in Mughal miniatures in India. But the methods of both the primitive artists and Matisse result in a loss of pictorial information on the volume of objects, which shadows cast by bodies on themselves (body shadows) can convey.

Medieval paintings were largely religious. But then, if paintings up to, say, the fifteenth century were divorced from reality, they would not be expected to be realistic. If they were not realistic, the illumination that they were seen in was unimportant as long as they conveyed a message and were visible. Many of them were produced at the behest of great ecclesiastics, usually to hang in churches, where lighting was frequently indifferent and often modified by the influence of stained glass which filtered daylight.

Because shadows imply direction, the lighting situation in churches would have been an additional discouragement: if a window were on the right of a painting and the shadows had been pointing toward it, the incongruity of the situation would have been obvious. That the early masters were aware of this is clear from Masacchio's pioneering mid-fourteenth-century frescoes about the Old Testament in the Brancacci chapel of Santa Maria delle Carmine in Florence. Though no shadow is shown to be cast on the ground, body shadows are in consonance with the fenestration of the church.

ADAPTATION

The term "adaptation" reflects a state of equilibrium of the nervous system. It represents essentially a state of readiness of the nervous system to respond to an appropriate stimulus. When the level of readiness is low, the stimulus has to be intense and vice versa. One of the early descriptions of adaptation appears in Dante's *Divine Comedy*. When Virgil conducts the poet through the underworld, and they come to a particularly putrid pit, the poet is revolted, but the Latin poet reassures him to the effect that, after a few moments, he will get used to the smell, and fail to perceive it.

In the visual sense, the term "adaptation" is frequently applied to distinguish between the adjustment to light and dark. As noted in Chapter 1, the retinal cones operate mainly in daylight, and the rods at low levels of illumination, with well-known consequences for the perception of detail and of colors. But this dichotomy represents a simplification. There exists a variety of states of light adaptation, contingent on the level of illumination and/or its tint. For example, if we gaze at a green surface for a little time and then direct our eyes at a grey or white one, our perception will be suffused by the complementary color, namely pink. The reason is that the retinal cones become adapted to green and thus are less sensitive to that color. Remember that Newton showed that white light is made up of all the colors of the rainbow. Therefore a green light reflected from the white or gray surface and imaged on a green-adapted retina would meet with a reduction in the retinal readiness to respond, with only the complementary colors being able to evoke a sensation.

This is where, pictorially speaking, shadows play a role. Intuitively, we associate well-defined, highly contrasted shadows with sunshine. Moonlight, too, gives rise to shadows, but our failure to discern sharp outlines at low illumination levels makes them appear fuzzy. An informed realistic artist will use this to good account and hint at the desired level of adaptation. However, his intention can be thwarted by the illumination later falling on his work. This is where the art historian must advise the lighting engineer: if possible, it is important to establish what environment any commissioned painting was intended for and to provide lighting that can fulfill the artist's objective.

This is no fanciful academic point. When Ghirlandaio, the endearing Florentine fifteenth-century artist, painted frescoes in Santa Maria Novella he took full account of the light coming through the colorful stained glass windows of the church, which he had himself provided in the interest of chromatic harmony.[1] He was not to know that one day the glass would be replaced with something bearing no coloristic resemblance to the original, thereby upsetting the chromatic balance of the frescoes.

The issue of adaptation and the pictorial representation of adaptational states is further exemplified by a consideration of nocturnes. Note that one can distinguish daylight from sunlight because only the latter gives rise to well-defined shadows. Night light stands apart in that colors are barely discernible, detail is wanting, and the level of illumination is obviously low. The paradox of viewing nocturnes in the flood of light provided in modern galleries is therefore glaring.

It is sometimes reasoned that painters show nocturnes but do not expect us to see them in the dark. This argument fails to take into account the very nature of adaptation. An example will make this clear. Ever since the Renaissance, paintings have been looked on as windows on the world. Suppose a painter produces a moonlit landscape. This is then ordinarily hung on a well-lit wall under daylight conditions. Next, suppose that you are in a country house. It is night, the moon is reflected from some lake or river below, and you want to see the view. If you stay well away from a window overlooking the water, and your room is brightly lit, you will see nothing. Switching off the room lights might be antisocial, but stepping near the window to avoid the light adaptation produced by the brightly lit walls of the room is not. Thus, the conflict between what the painter wants to show us and what the director of the picture gallery permits is real.

Two of the first nocturnes to have been painted are in the form of miniatures found in an illuminated manuscript, the *Trés Riches Heures du Duc de Berry*, executed by the Limbourg brothers (1420). They depict the darkness at the time of the crucifixion and Gethsemane. As they appear in a book, there can be no question of our adaptation being controlled by either miniature, the color of the paper being the overriding determinant. As a sort of concession to color changes in the dark, the pictures are executed in cool (bluish) and warm (olive) tones of gray (Fig. 7-2). It is noteworthy that the sky is dark blue, and trees are shown in a somber green. Note that the sixteenth-century natural philosopher Lord Bacon had anticipated the duplicity theory of vision when, long after the Limbourg brothers had departed this life, he said (in a religious context) that "all colours agree in the dark."[2] A similar observation obviously cannot have escaped the Limbourg brothers since they toned down their colors. But they did not quite believe their eyes, for it is not what they observed in the dark that they painted but what they thought was there.

Clear evidence of a profound understanding of the nature of visual adaptation is provided by one of the greatest painters of the Italian Renaissance, Piero della Francesca (1417?-1492). It will suffice for our purpose to confine our attention to two of his works. The first is the predella of his large Virgin with child and saints polyptych, now in the National Gallery in Perugia. Recall that however recondite the theological content of an altar piece, the predella underneath consists of several small paintings with messages for the unlearned and untutored multitude.

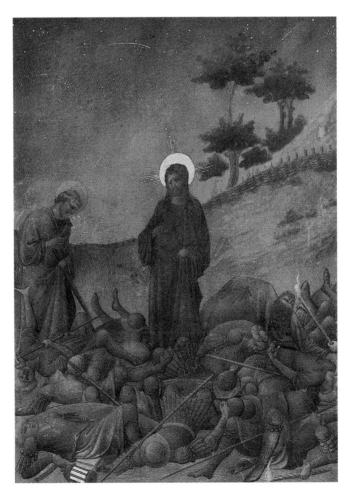

FIGURE 7-2

Limbourg Brothers. *Christ in the Garden of Olives, Trés Riches Heures du Duc de Berry.*
(Musée Conde, Chantilly, France. Giraudon/Art Resource, NY.)

The component of the St. Francis predella that differs from the other two colored ones is the central one which depicts the stigmatization of the saint (Fig. 7-3). It appears in an eerie light. So peculiar is its effect that, in the words of Murray and de Vecchi,, "Christ's light seems to cover [the surrounding landscape] with snow."[3] The reason for this is plain: the stigmatization is seen in too much light. When, for want of a better way of conducting the relevant crucial experiment, we view a color reproduction in semidarkness, the mystery is resolved and turns into mysteriousness: what is insinuated is a scene illuminated by moonlight, and, for all we know, it is in such light that Piero painted this panel. We have to remember that, until our own vandal-ridden days, places of worship never closed. If, during the night, a disturbed soul went to seek solace in front of the polyptych, the colors would be silent. But one panel would speak to the orant, for he or she would see it realistically in a way in which poorly lit scenes would have appeared to the dark-adapted eye in those times of sparse artificial lighting.

The other example of Piero's insight into the problem of adaptation is more complex and sophisticated. It is provided by his frescoes in the church of San Francesco in Arezzo. The two that concern us here are *Dream of Constantine* (Fig. 7-4) and *Battle of Constantine and Maxentius* (Fig. 7-5). The former depicts the emperor at night, prostrate on his couch, watched over by his bodyguard, while the angel prophesying victory dives like a bird of prey above the canvas of the tent. It is painted on a wall that never receives direct sunlight, and it is unestablished whether Piero painted by the light of a full moon. The colors are faint, insinuating moonlight, and contrast with the diurnal illumination, introduced in a second fresco, which shows the battle on the following day. Constantine is shown on horse-back: with his army behind him, and the diminutive cross of his dream in front of him, he rides against the turning and defeated host on his right. From the religious point of view, the figure of the victorious emperor provides the link between the two scenes.

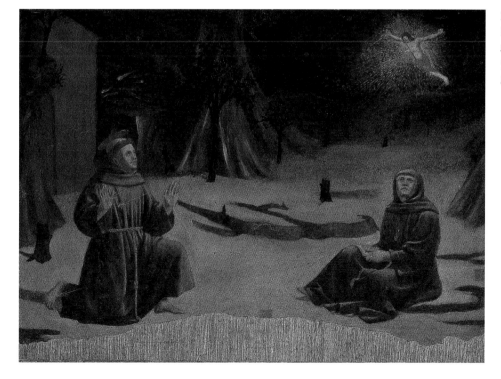

FIGURE   7-3

Piero della Francesca. *Predella with St. Francis Receiving the Stigmata.*
(Galleria Nazionale dell'Umbria, Perugia, Italy. Scala/Art Resource, NY.)

FIGURE 7-4

Piero della Francesca. *The Story of the True Cross: The Dream of Constantine.*

(S. Francesco, Arezzo, Italy. Scala/Art Resource, NY.)

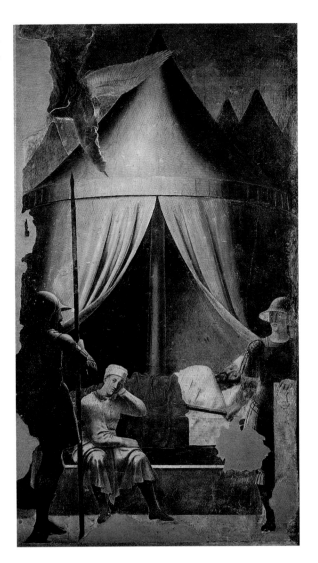

But for Piero, the innovator and rebel, the link between the two is found in the rendering of the emperor's bodyguard. Ignored by writers who have concerned themselves with this sublime Tuscan artist,[4,5,6] he appears in *Battle* on the emperor's left, a helmeted man, also on horseback. Unquestioningly obedient, as all of his ilk have been at the state's behest, this member of the imperial bodyguard is first in one respect. Piero shows him with a sharp shadow of a helmet bisecting his Italian face (see Fig. 7-5) and invites comparison with the same face shown in *Dream*. It would appear that this is the earliest example of a realistic rendering of an obviously sun-drenched scene painted in this millenium.

We should not leave this topic without placing it in its cultural context. It is easy to show that cast shadows begin to reappear in European painting only after the middle of the fifteenth century, the date of the above works. Remember that, within Piero's memory, artists had been painting light as though they were painting God. Piero painted different levels of adaptation because he was able to paint his understanding of the seen world without having to put it into words, and because papal understanding of visual physiology was even poorer than that of later cosmology, Piero was saved the ignominy faced by Galileo. Yet this does not mean that his offense was any the smaller; he was, after all, the first to convey the notion that light resides not in God but in the eye.

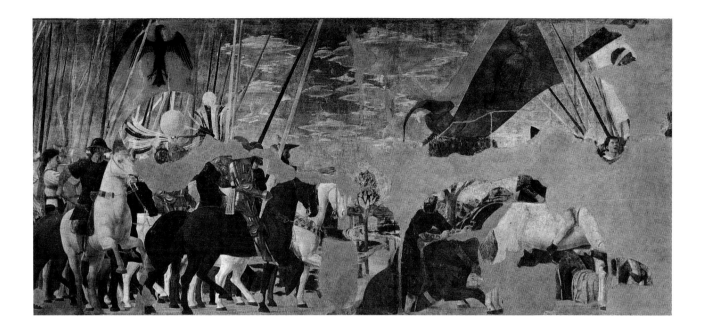

LIGHT BRAVURAS

The next 50 years witnessed that the fraternity of pictorial artists had begun to assimilate realistically the rendering of adaptational effects and shadows. Five centuries later it is amusing to note the hesitancy with which this was being achieved, as though they were naughty children and tried their hardest not to be caught. There were numerous examples to show this. Mair from Landshut produced a woodcut called *The Nativity* in 1499 (Fig. 7-6). He rendered a very credible shadow of the leg of what appears to be the messenger in the bottom left corner, but note how the shadow of Joseph's walking stick terminates incomplete. *An Annunciation* by Fra Angelico (1400-1455) and St. Jerome in his *Study by Carpaccio* (1502?) both show a similarly shy restraint. And, though Caravaggio (1573-1610) seems to have been the first artist to record the sundial effect (Fig. 7-7), which appears when a painter renders different objects at different times of the day and natural daylight changes the direction whereby they are illuminated so that the various shadows point in different directions, problems persisted for centuries. Note the baroque swing of the (second) portrait of Colonel van Heythuysen by the great Dutch portraitist Frans Hals (1637?). What are we to make of the shadow of the stool the soldier is balancing on (Fig. 7-8)? The only rational reading of this peculiar construct is based on the supposition that somewhere underneath the colonel's backside there burned a candle—upside down.

As artists came to terms with shadows, they also attempted to render a variety of types of illumination in the same painting. This is a dauntingly demanding problem with respect to adaptation, and it has never been noted as a feature of the Renaissance, perhaps because the pioneering steps were taken not in Italy but north of the Alps by the greatly underestimated Danube artist Albrecht Altdorfer (1480?-1520).

This burger of Ratisbon, a graphic artist and a painter in oils, is said to have been the first to have painted the sun. During his life, the horizon of the world was rapidly expanding: his life coincided with the multiplication of vast voyages, and Christopher Columbus was his contemporary. An analogous expansion of a painter's vision into wider and wider space cannot therefore come altogether as a surprise.

FIGURE 7-5

Piero della Francesca. *Battle of Constantine and Maxentius. From The Story of the True Cross.*

(S. Francesco, Arezzo, Italy. Scala/Art Resource, NY.)

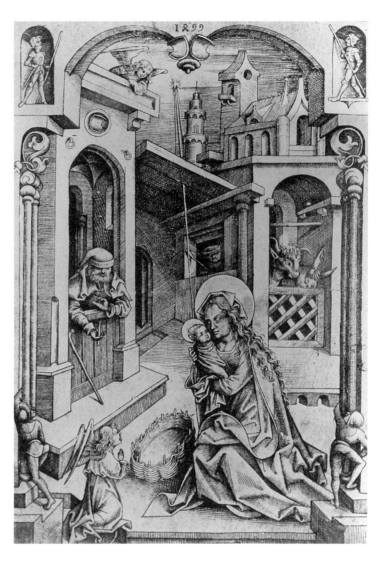

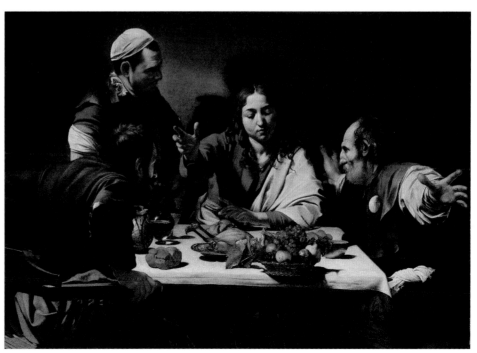

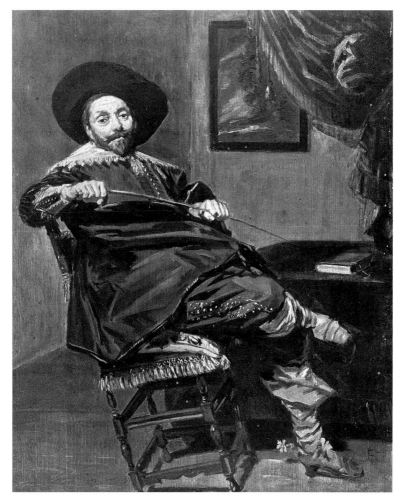

FIGURE 7-8
Hals. *Portrait de Willem van Heythuysen.*
(Musées royaux des Beaux-Arts de Belgique, Bruxelles-Koninklijke Musea voor Schone Kunsten van België, Brussels.)

Two panels from Altdorfer's altarpiece, originally painted for the Austrian St. Florian monastery near Linz on the Danube, and still on view there, illustrate his handling of the effects of different lighting in one place. Not until the seventeenth century can one find a departure from the rule valid for Altdorfer, as it was for Raphael, Vasari and other artists, that multiple types of light source were introduced in the rendering of supernatural events of heightened emotional content. This is what Altdorfer illustrates with *Agony in the Garden of Olives* and *The Arrest of Jesus*.

Figure 7-9 shows Jesus, getting down on his knees in front of the angel holding the cup of bitterness who appears in a cutting in a rock. A man in the middle distance holds a torch, and a German township stretches across the background of the scene. Lit by glancing rays of the setting sun, a hillock and a mountain rise behind the town with a hidden moon overhead. The vermilion sky above the bluish mountain offers a pattern of chromatic contrast (which Delacroix was later to believe to have originated with Raphael).

This raises the problem of coloristic realism, and two points are to be noted. In the first place, the illumination by the overhead moonlight is coded with a cool white as in Piero della Francesca's earlier *Dream of Constantine*. Though Altdorfer had visited Italy at least once, there is no evidence that he had reached as far south as Arezzo: Venice tended to be the mecca of German artists at that time. Altdorfer realistically chilled his highlights, but, unlike Piero, he failed to desatu-

FIGURE   7-9
**Atldorfer. *Agony in the
Garden of Olives.***
From the Saint Sebastian altar, 1518.
*(Abbey of St. Florian. Erich Lessing/
Art Resource, NY.)*

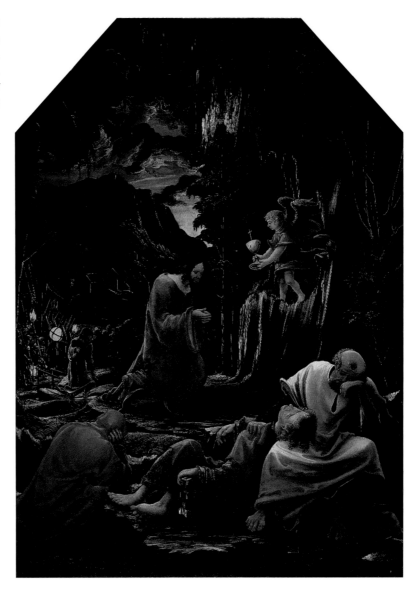

rate his colors, fresh even today. We have already noted that color vision deteriorates even when the moon is full, and there is no question that colors can be seen with the glow with which Altdorfer endows them. The dilemma he found himself in is neatly epitomized by the setting sun licking the sides of the houses in the town, which act like barriers separating the light of the sun from that of the moon. The difficulty of artificially illuminating such a painting so as to create a realistic impression is manifest because if the (artificial) illumination matches one of the illuminants, it will fail with the other.

This is also true of *Saint Peter Cuts off the Ear of Malchus*, which is one of the most ambitious works ever painted with respect to illumination (Fig. 7-10). It far surpasses Altdorfer's *Agony in the Garden of Olives* while illustrating the insurmountable difficulties that this problem presents. As before, and as is inevitable if both sun and moonlight are to appear, the setting sun reddens the distant sky while the foreground is illuminated by the moon. Altdorfer achieves this with cool pizzicato strokes reflected from the soldier's armor and helmets; from the folds of Christ's red cloak; and from St. Peter's bald head, yellow cloak, and drawn sword

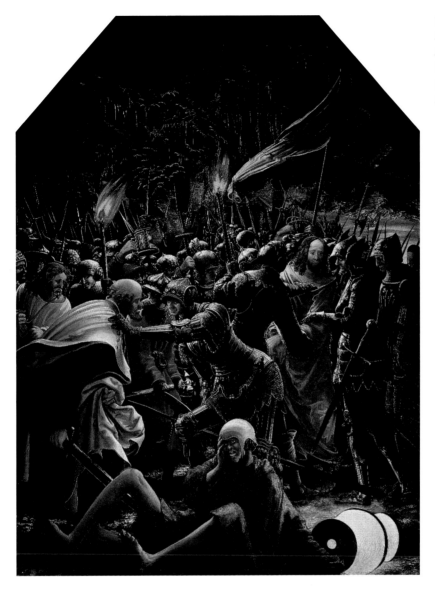

FIGURE   7-10

Altdorfer. *Saint Peter Cuts Off the Ear of Malchus.*

From the Saint Sebastian altar, 1518. *(Abbey of St. Florian. Erich Lessing/Art Resource, NY.)*

with which the apostle has just cut off the left ear of the unfortunate Malchus. The colors of the cloaks are just as intense as in *Agony in the Garden of Olives*, but the torches provide some measure of credibility with regard to chromatic tone.

Rafael's *Liberation of St. Peter* in the Stanza d'Eliodoro in the Vatican, painted some 10 years earlier (1524), magnifies the adaptational difficulty (Fig. 7-11). The reason is that it attempts to set up a relation among four types of light: (1) light from the setting sun, as reflected from the clouds below; (2) the quarter crescent moon; (3) a torch held by one of the Roman soldiers; and (4) depictions of two nonphysical lights emanating from the angel rescuing the apostle.

There is no way to illuminate this fresco so as to present realistic tonal values. The nimbus surrounding the angel is golden, and recalls sunlight. The scant lighting in the Stanza d'Eliodore serves to disguise the resultant pictorial inconsistencies. The worldly (physical) lights appear exclusively on the left, and the reflections from armor which were also to baffle Altdorfer make it difficult to decide whether the two guards asleep across the path of liberation are lit by the angel or the moon.

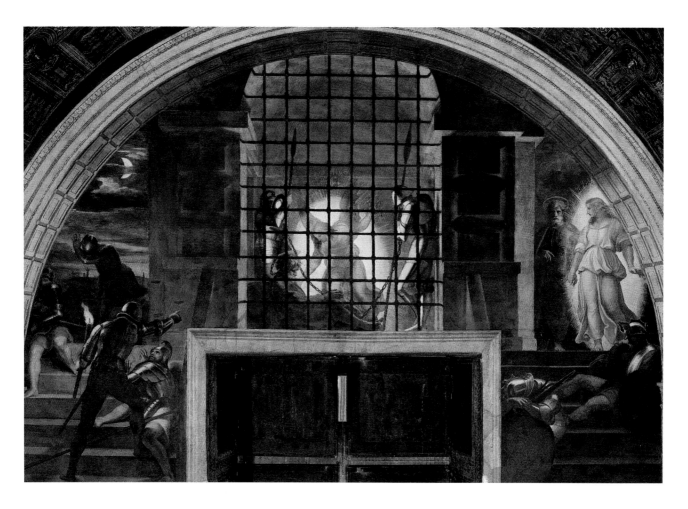

ADAPTATION OUTWITTED?

It was Rembrandt (1606-1669) who first produced work free from vacillation insofar as different types of light is concerned. He lived in a milieu of skepticism, and, though a Mennonite, as a contemporary of Huygens and of Spinoza, he would not have been unacquainted with the rigors of intellectual analysis. He did not evade the challenge of rendering light that may have been extraterrestrial: in the painting of Danae, now destroyed, he showed the radiance emanating from silver as though the metal were a source of light. Moreover, he managed to avoid the inconsistencies of earlier artists. This is exemplified in a number of paintings, as in *The Descent from the Cross in Munich*, but *Belshazzar's Feast* (Fig. 7-12) provides far and away the best insight into his understanding.

Only Bode[7] seems to have addressed the drama of Rembrandt's solution of an interesting psychological problem, namely that of Banquo coming to the feast and being seen by Macbeth alone.

No one but Belshazzar sees the writing on the wall. As if to press this point home, Rembrandt has his guests illuminated by unseen roomlights, clearly and systematically reflected in the corneae of their eyes. The reflections do not show the writing on the wall but a source on our left. The writing is self-luminous and lights up the king's face. There is no biblical authority (Dan. 5:5) for the nature of the characters. Like most writing, it could have been black, but then it would have

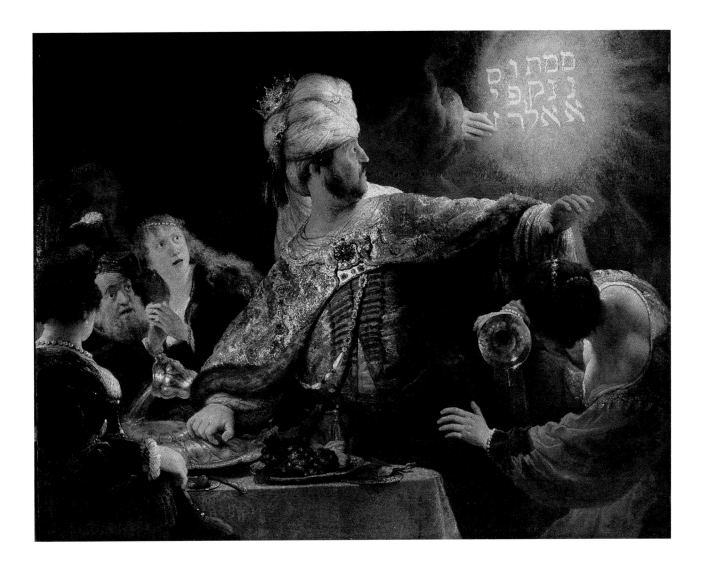

FIGURE   7-12

Rembrandt. *Belshazzar's Feast.*

(Reproduced by courtesy of the Trustees, The National Gallery, London.)

hardly attracted the king's attention. There is no mention of the fiery characters seen by Bode: in any case, fire would not have made for legibility. but phosphorescence would have been known in any Dutch household where fish was eaten. Fish bones can be seen to phosphoresce in the dark, and it is in cold phosphorescent light that the writing appears. Because the letters throw their light, even if only as a metaphor, solely on the king, they do not have to compete with the ambient illumination on the rest of the canvas, and the above-mentioned difficulties of Renaissance artists are eschewed.

The painting is almost a nocturne, and the full light in which the National Gallery exhibits it today is desirable from the standpoint of those wishing to examine the minutiae of the design. But the surfeit of the illumination detracts from the drama and all but muzzles the mystery. If it were shown in more appropriate conditions, Belshazzar would be seen like a bird hovering in the air, suspended between the writing and a table, where his right hand provides the only formal link with his boon companions in that it rests at the center of the semicircle which they describe.

FIGURE 7-13
Rembrandt. *The Artist's Studio.*
(Ashmolean Museum, Oxford.)

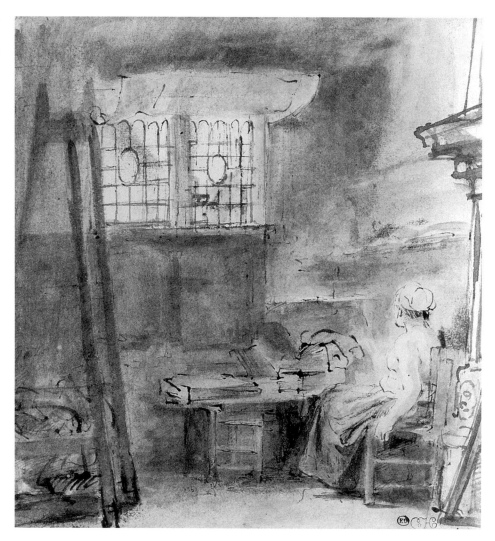

A RETURN TO THE NORTH

Caravaggio, the inventor of chiaroscuro (a representation of light and dark without regard to color) presents no adaptational dilemma. His scenes rarely distinguish between indirect or cloudy light and direct sunlight; where there are shadows they are realistic (see Fig. 7-7), and many of his works are found in poorly lit places so that the very invention of chiaroscuro appears as almost mandatory. In fact, he provided the only pictorially feasible answer to the ecclesiastic darkness in which many of the paintings of those days were enshrined. He liberated realistic illumination, though it is just as well to note that chiaroscuro paintings look more realistic in subdued rather than broad light. Caravaggio provided a sort of rule-of-thumb defense against a lack of understanding of the admittedly difficult principles of visual adaptation.

He found imitators in Southern Italy and in Spain, but the developers of his ideas were in the north. It was not unusual for northern artists to spend a few years in Rome. However, there is no evidence that either Georges De la Tour or Rembrandt ever went south, and their caravaggiste concern with light is almost certainly derived via intermediaries.

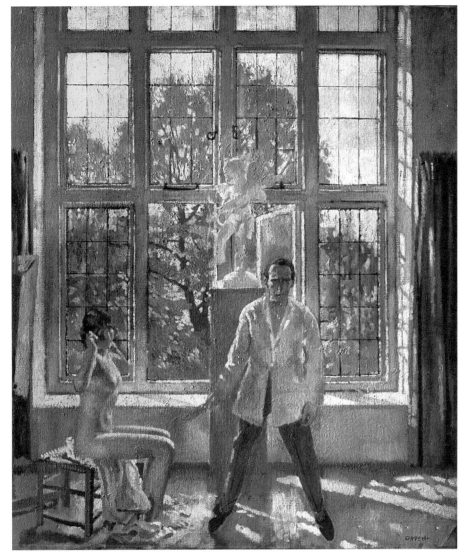

FIGURE 7-14

Orpen. *Summer Afternoon (The Artist in His Studio with a Model).*

(Bequest of John T. Spaulding. Courtesy, Museum of Fine Arts, Boston.)

De la Tour presents an all-or-none situation: his oeuvre consists of scenes illuminated by daylight or artificial light. Whether or not the paintings actually represent the output of two different artists, like father and son, is a matter for art historians.[8] As noted earlier, with respect to van Honthorst's *Christ before the High Priest*, De la Tour's nocturnal scenes demand more illumination with warmer light than do those showing daylight.

It may be instructive, at this point, to digress and to inquire into the conditions in which artists painted. Breughel (1525-1569) was among the early artists to show an artist at work, and others have gone so far as to indicate a schematized layout of their studio. A comparison of Adriaen van Ostade's (1610-1685) renderings of his studios is instructive. The one in the Rijksmuseum in Amsterdam shows a small window on the left, and the artist is shown painting a rocky landscape. The presumably later painting (1663) in Dresden suggests that he has moved to affluent quarters: the window here is much larger with more light getting into the studio, a powerful pointer this for those who may be tempted to overemphasize the significance of changes in an artist's style.

FIGURE 7-15
Whistler. *Old Battersea Bridge (Nocturne in Blue and Silver).*
*(Tate Gallery, London. Erich Lessing/
Art Resource, NY.)*

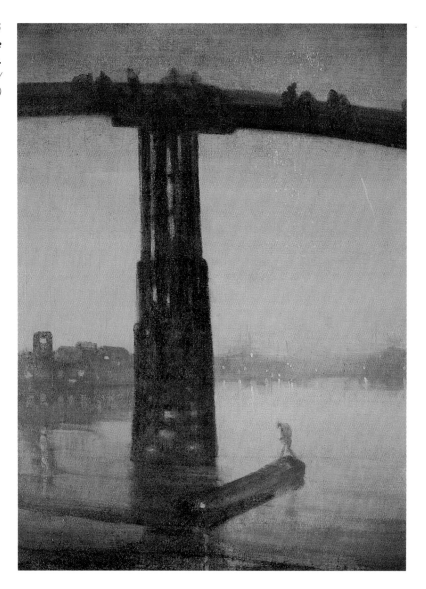

The pen-and-brush drawing by Rembrandt (1655/1656) shows a small studio with a small, high-up window, faced by a nude model, the impression created being almost that of a prison cell rather than of a place of work (Fig. 7-13). This provides insight into Rembrandt's type of chiaroscuro, for it is evident that, even if his sitter received an adequate amount of light, the background must have been dark, as is true of most of his portraits. This helps to explain why the appearance of his portraits is relatively insensitive to the type of illumination in which they are exhibited. The dark surrounds insulate tone and color from a potentially hostile photic environment, be it a vulgar gilt frame or inappropriate ambient illumination.

In the nineteenth century, artists' studios became well lit, perhaps because windows even in bourgeois houses had become larger. Sir William Orpen's *Summer Afternoon (The Artist in His Studio with a Model)* is a case in point. Unlike Rembrandt in the above-mentioned drawing, this painter (1878-1931) is evidently more interested in himself than in the model (Fig. 7-14): the studio is suffused with sunlight entering through windows reaching the ceiling, and both model and easel seem mere incidentals, separated by an open window from the central confident self-portraitist.

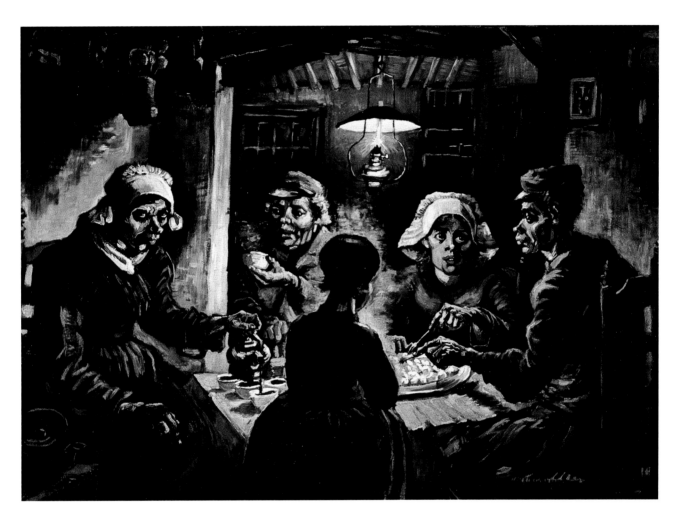

PERCEIVED TWILIGHT

It is not surprising that light as a sensation became understood only during the second half of the nineteenth century. Great strides forward had been made in the understanding of the physiology and psychology of vision. In their own ways, both Turner and Seurat had tried to paint in light of the scientific principles as they understood them (see Chapters 8 and 11). Photography was making an impact, giving rise to the first wave of photo-realism, as exemplified in the meticulous portraits and still lifes of Fantin-Latour. Additionally, domestic artificial lighting levels had been raised following the introduction of gaslight and the invention of the brilliantly luminous Welsbach mantle. The last hurdles in the depiction of light, or rather its dearth and absence, were soon taken.

Whistler's *Old Battersea Bridge* (Fig. 7-15) provides one example of dearth of light and van Gogh's *Potato Eaters* (Fig. 7-16) another. The first impression created by the American's painting (1872?) is one of an unaccustomed perspective: a gigantic T spreads across the canvas, and, high up, silhouetted against the trisected sky, there are profiles of people in umpteen different postures. But we should have been alerted to the artist's intention by reading the title in full. The location is preceded by a description of the genre, namely *Nocturne in Blue and Silver*. Night is rapidly falling on the proximal side of the foreground; color and detail have vanished. Silver contrasts with darkness to accentuate tonality, and the indefiniteness of Impressionism lends itself to imitate that of vision in the dark.

FIGURE 7-16

Van Gogh. *The Potato Eaters.*

(Amsterdam, Van Gogh Museum [Vincent van Gogh Foundation].)

In the case of van Gogh, we have the rare benefit of an artist commenting on what he did and why. Writing to his brother Theo in 1885 about the genesis of his oil painting *The Potato Eaters* (Fig. 7-16) (he had also produced a lithograph of the same scene), he says that he had started painting it by daylight but finished by artificial light, presumably by that of an oil lamp imaged in the middle of the canvas, much as van Honthorst had done with a candle. This letter proves beyond any shadow of doubt that van Gogh had no desire to "correct" a seminocturnal painting so that it might look convincing in daylight. On the contrary, he had started to paint in daylight and was, as he states in his letter, dissatisfied. Later touches were therefore added under the lighting conditions under which he had perceived the scene. If ever justification was needed to show that good exhibiting may require ad hoc illumination, then van Gogh has provided it.

But each painting must be judged on its own. In a letter van Gogh wrote in 1888 relating to his painting *The Night Cafe* (see Fig. 10-1) he describes how "for three nights running I sat up to paint and went to bed during the day. I often think the night is more alive and more richly coloured than the day. . . . I have tried to express the terrible passions of humanity by means of red and green. The room is blood red and dark yellow with a green billiard table in the middle; there are four lemon yellow lamps with a glow of orange and green."[9] In this case the nocturnal nature of the painting is accidental: the dark serves to accentuate the colors, and the impact of the painting would be reduced if seen in less than bright artificial illumination.

PHOTIC CORRECTNESS

There are some practical conclusions to be drawn from the above considerations. The galleries of the world present paintings as though these were to be arranged in a visual catalogue. Given the organization of professional training—for the history of art is seen as a part of history in general—the division of paintings is by period and by country. This explains why paintings are grouped together in "schools." Some schools are larger than others, and a Rembrandt nocturnal Nativity has been known to hang next to a swirling sea-scape by van de Veldte, because both belong to the Dutch school. Such an oft-repeated arrangement is nothing more or less than a visual solecism.

That said, it is self-evident that providing the ideal canvas-oriented lighting would be prohibitively expensive. We shall return to the matter after discussing a simple experiment that should demonstrate that gallery lighting and our eyes create problems for the appreciation of paintings.

In one of Leonardo's notebooks he describes the use of what may be conveniently referred to as a peashooter. That artist had some peculiar ideas about the formation of the retinal image and about magnification.[10] For instance, he claimed that when one looks at a scene through a tube the image appears larger than to the bare eye. It is just possible that as a result of the reduction of stray light striking the retina, Leonardo may have found the image clearer and interpreted this as larger. But the point to bear in mind here is that the appearance of paintings can be changed when one looks through a tube. Indeed, looking through one formed by one's balled fist can lead to a dramatic intensification of colors, even in highly chromatic pictures, and to a revelation of a change in atmosphere in nocturnal ones. It is important to maintain such a viewing distance as to obscure the wall surface surrounding the canvas in view. This demonstrates that the adaptational and corollary effects resulting from well-lit walls materially affect our perceptions. It further shows that the ambient illumination in galleries, particularly when they are lit from above, may adulterate viewing and interfere with the artist's message.

It should now be obvious that there is a real conflict between the illumination policy of great galleries and the needs of the observing eye. It is cheaper to illuminate canvases with natural or artificial light if it is distributed more or less randomly, but this method is counterproductive for the reasons stated above. It might be possible to devise screening that would allow the walls to be lit and the onlookers' eyes shaded, but here again the cost-benefit ratio may prove to be an obstacle except perhaps in very special conditions. For example, *The Mona Lisa* in the Louvre is now protected not only by armed guards but also by an enclosure that renders it all but invisible. It has been reduced to an icon which to have passed by is counted as a privilege.

However, some improvements are surely possible at a manageable cost. From the point of view of visual appreciation, the knot tying together different components of a school and including photically diverse elements should be cut. Nocturnes and scenes stipulating viewing in low levels of adaptation should be gathered in a part of even a large hall, segregated from others needing plenty of light, and the light shed on them judiciously reduced. This simple attention to ophthalmic fundamentals would transform the enjoyment attainable from across the ages, and also from contemporary works of art.

— REFERENCES —

1. Brown JW: *The Dominican Church of Santa Maria Novella at Florence*, Otto Schulze, Edinburgh, Scotland, 1902.
2. Quoted in Devey J: *Lord Bacon's Essays*, George Bell, London, 1888, p. 10.
3. Murray P., de Vecchi P: *Piero della Francesca*, Weidenfeld & Nicolson, London, 1970, p. 104.
4. Hendy P: *Piero della Francesca and the Early Renaissance*, Weidenfeld & Nicholson, London, 1968.
5. Clark K: *Piero della Francesca*, Phaidon, London, 1951.
6. Longhi R: *Piero della Francesca*, GC Sansoni, Firenze, Italy, 1963.
7. Bode W: *Rembrandt*, Charles Sedelmayer, Paris, 1897.
8. Wright C: *Masters of Candle-light*, Arcos-Verlag, Landshut, Germany, 1995.
9. The Complete Letters of Vincent van Gogh ed 2: New York Graphic Society, Greenwich, Conn., 1959. Letter 533.
10. Weale R: Leonardo and the eye, *Doc Ophthalmol* 68:19-34, 1988.

Part Four

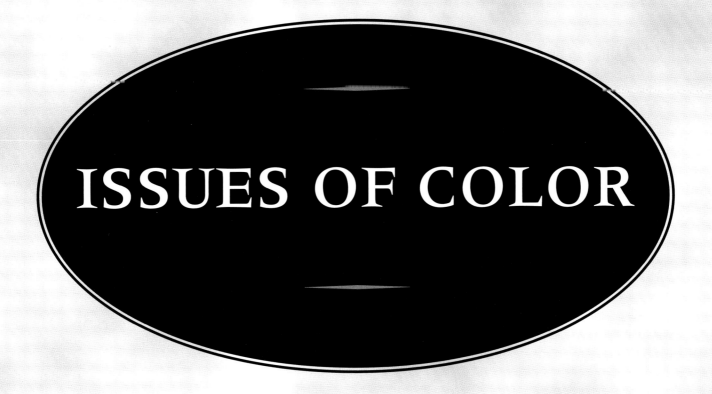

ISSUES OF COLOR

Chapter Eight

A CIRCLE OF COLOR

TURNER, NEWTON, AND GOETHE

Michael F. Marmor

The nature of color has intrigued scientists, philosophers, and artists through-out history. Modern science has elucidated the physical nature of light and reconciled the quantum and wave natures of electromagnetic radiation. However, the mechanisms by which physical stimuli are translated into the subjective perception of color are still subjects of study and debate. Schools of art today teach about light and color, but there is no universally accepted color circle, and in art the physiologic effects of using and juxtaposing colors are difficult to separate from the cultural and psychologic impact of colors. This situation is not so different from that 200 years ago when J.M.W. Turner (1775-1851) was a young artist, evaluating the science and theory of the day, and formulating his ideas about color and style.

Isaac Newton (1642-1727) was already very famous by Turner's time, more than 100 years after Newton's seminal discovery that white light is broken by a prism into a full spectrum of colors. Newton had interpreted this observation to indicate that white light is a mixture of all the spectral colors, and he argued that light was therefore corpuscular in nature, a concept that could not be fully verified until the advent of quantum mechanics. This was counterintuitive to those who accepted the Aristotelian belief that color was not a property of light but rather a feature of visible objects.[1] They reasoned that, since color was not visible without light, it followed that color was a feature of each object and appeared only upon interaction with light (which itself had no color). This logic was hard to shake, even in the face of Newton's experiments, and debate over these issues raged for nearly 2 centuries.[2] Newton's supporters during this period praised him lavishly, and made him a national hero. Many popular accounts of his work appeared (much as current books explain the theory of relativity), including *Newtonianism for Ladies*. Voltaire popularized Newton in France with *Elémens de la Philosophie de Neuton*. Alexander Pope glorified Newton in a famous couplet:

> Nature, and Nature's Laws lay hid in Night.
> God said, *Let Newton be*! and All was Light.[2]

On the other hand, even reputable scientists like Huygens and Hooke criticized Newton's theory where it failed to explain the wavelike properties of light. Bishop Berkeley took offense at Newton's science as a threat to theology. And Samuel Taylor Coleridge feared that Newton's scientific rigor corrupted the imagination: "I believe the souls of five hundred Sir Isaac Newtons would go to the making up of a Shakespeare or a Milton."[2]

Wolfgang von Goethe (1749-1832) was among those, in this time of intellectual turmoil, who had trouble accepting Newton's concept that white light was divisible into colors. Goethe is most famous as a poet and playwright and as author of *Faust*, which is arguably one of the great literary masterpieces of all time. But Goethe, a true Renaissance man, was also famous in his time as a philosopher and scientist. He wrote a highly regarded book on botany, was the first to recognize a bony feature of the skull, and he both named and founded the scientific discipline of "morphology."[3] He was interested in phenomenon of perception and carried out many careful observational experiments about colors and how they are perceived. In 1810 he published a book called *Theory of Colours*[4] which incorporated his scientific observations and his philosophy about the perception of color, along with a rather pointed and at times polemical refutation of Newton's corpuscular theory of light. Goethe's work has been largely disregarded in modern times, since Newton's physical observations about light have proven accurate. However, Goethe's book was well received and widely read in its own time, particularly by those who still questioned Newton and by artists or philosophers who were more interested in the sensory than physical aspects of color. No less a figure than Beethoven said, "Can you lend me *The Theory of Colors* for a few weeks? It is an important work. His last things are insipid."[5]

Turner grew up amidst these scientific developments and controversies. He could not help but be aware of Newton's work, although we have no evidence that he specifically read or contemplated Newton's reports on color. We know that Turner lectured for many years about color as well as other aspects of art as part of his duties as professor of perspective at the Royal Academy and that he referred his students in one lecture to a Newtonian account of the formation of colors.[6] We also know that he owned a copy of the English translation of Goethe's *Theory of Colours*, which was published in 1840, late in Turner's life. He read it carefully and made extensive marginal notes that give some insight as to how Turner interpreted the great playwright's musings about color theory and color perception.[7]

Turner trained as an architect in his youth, but his extraordinary skill in drawing soon became apparent and he was admitted to the art school of the Royal Academy. Within a few years his pictures were on display and by his mid-20s he was elected to full membership in the academy. In 1807 he was appointed professor of perspective, a post that he held for many years. He diligently prepared a course of lectures, and even planned a book (which was never written), to teach his approach to art. Contemporaries, however, describe him as a remarkably

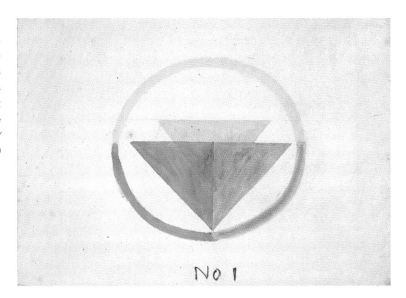

FIGURE 8-1
Turner. *Watercolor Circle.
No. 1.* c. 1818. This diagram empha-
sizes the primary pigment colors
(red, yellow, and blue) and shows
how yellow is used to represent
light, while red and blue below are
shadow. (*Tate Gallery, London/
Art Resource, N.Y.*)

obscure speaker.[8] One wrote "You could hardly hear anything Turner said, he rambled on in a very indistinct way which was most difficult to follow. . . . But though the subject matter of his lectures was neither listened to nor understood, they were well attended as he used to display beautiful drawings of imaginary buildings with fine effects of light and shade." Another wrote, "Turner's lectures on perspective, from his naturally enigmatical and ambiguous style of delivery, were almost unintelligible. Half of each lecture was addressed to the attendant behind him, who was constantly busied, under his muttered directions, in selecting from a huge portfolio drawings and diagrams to illustrate his teaching. Many of these were truly beautiful, speaking intelligibly enough to the eye if his language did not to the ear."

Although Turner took his lectures seriously, and made detailed notes of his material, he didn't deliver his first lectures until 1811, 4 years after he was appointed professor of perspective, and he gave lectures only sporadically thereafter. That he may have had some unconscious ambivalence about teaching is illustrated by a series of incidents before his 1814 lectures.[9] The first lecture on January 3 was canceled because he left his demonstration portfolio in the hackney coach on the way to the Royal Academy. Turner advertised in the *Morning Chronicle* for its return, and the finder advertised as well (although with a dim view of their worth): "PORTFOLIO FOUND. . . containing some drawings on the Science of Perspective. . . . Should no application be made within fourteen days they will be disposed of as waste paper, being considered of little value." Turner's lecture was then rescheduled for 8:00 P.M. on January 10, but he did not appear at the scheduled time. When he finally arrived at 9:00, "in searching his pocket he ascertained that he had lost his lecture! . . . He had left the lecture in the hackney coach which had conveyed him." For the record, he did finally deliver the lecture—but 4 years later he again left his papers on a coach.

Turner's lecture notes show that he viewed color as subsidiary to light and dark, which were to him the most powerful elements of painting. The color circles he made to show in his lectures (Fig. 8-1) are based strongly on the primary paint colors of red, yellow, and blue, which dominated Turner's work throughout his career (Figs. 8-2 and 8-3). He wrote in his lecture notes, "suppose the yellow triangle light, red and blue shade" to emphasize that the dichotomy of light and dark was dominant over the colors. But then he gave meaning to the colors and said, "Hence we have gray morning, the yellow mid-day and crimson evening."

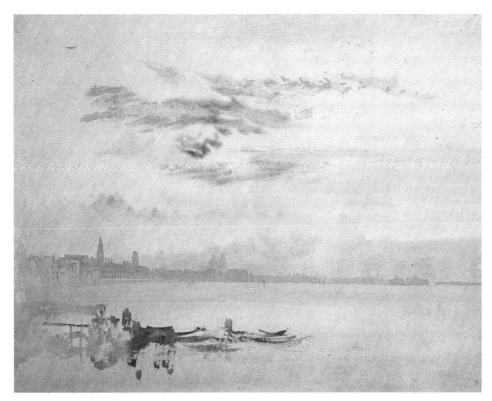

FIGURE 8-2
Turner. *Venice Looking East from the Giudecca.*
Watercolor, 1819. This impressionistic view is dominated, as many of Turner's works, by yellow light against blue water, with red adding a sense of drama. *(Tate Gallery, London/ Art Resource, NY.)*

Furthermore, "Green [is] the weakest of the direct rays," while "the strongest ray as to power, [is] red."[10] Indeed, throughout Turner's work, one sees a juxtaposition of yellow symbolizing light, blue indicating calmness and cold, and red as a throbbing power that selectively intercedes. Greens are used sparingly, if at all. Light and dark are usually the dominant forces to contend with, whether as a brilliant sun over the water, or as the darkening gloom of a storm.

Turner's powerful but selective use of colors did not go unnoticed by the critics of his time.[11] One wrote in 1827 of his picture *Mortlake Terrace* (see Fig. 1-28): "That the Lord Mayor's barge, which was introduced only for the sake of the colour, should look yellow in its gingerbread decorations, is natural; and that the Aldermen's wives should look yellow from sea-sickness is also natural. But that the trees should look yellow, that the Moffatt family themselves and all their friends and connections; dogs, grass plots and white stone copings of red brick walls should all be afflicted with the jaundice, is too much to be endured." Another critic speculated sarcastically in 1831 on whether it might be "disease (opthalmia [sic] or calenture [violent tropical fever and delirium]) which leads him into the most marvellous absurdities and audacities of colour that painter ever ventured on." A respected ophthalmologist, Liebreich, argued quite seriously[12] that Turner's use of reddish and yellow tones increased as he aged and might therefore be a result of developing cataract.

However, Turner's predisposition to yellow, as the color of light and day, began early in his career, long before one could possibly postulate eye disease. At age 23, his work was considered "too much to the brown" by a colleague; he was only 31 when a well-known collector Sir George Beaumont commented that "his colouring has become jaundiced."[13] Furthermore, even in Turner's late paintings, one finds representational details that could not have been done by an individual with significantly impaired sight. Yellow has fascinated many other artists, such as van Gogh (see Chapter 10), and we need not stretch medical probability to

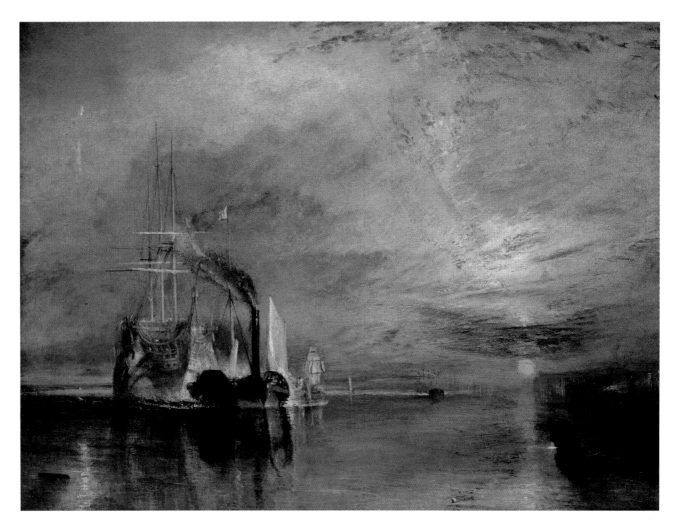

explain the artistic choice. With respect to the hazy images in Turner's works, the question of whether he was myopic is similar to that raised about Impressionism (see Chapter 3). Turner clearly could paint precise and representational works when he wished, and he included great detail in some later works, as we have noted; yet many of his pictures revel in the hazy light of dawn or mist. Spectacles were readily available in Turner's day, and there is no reason to think that he would not avail himself of good vision if he needed them. Some of his reading glasses have been preserved and have powers of +3.00 and +4.00 diopter, which indicates that he used spectacles when necessary and also that he was neither myopic nor severely farsighted.[14]

About the time that Turner was appointed professor at the Royal Academy of Art, Goethe was working on his book on color vision. He was deeply invested in this book, which linked color to his philosophical approach to the arts. Whether through error or pride, he chose to attack Newton as the source of error in color theory, and he did not mince words. He wrote that "a great mathematician was possessed with an entirely false notion on the physical origin of colors; yet, owing to his great authority as a geometer, the mistakes which he committed as an experimentalist long became sanctioned in the eyes of a world ever fettered in prejudices."[15] He refused to accept Newton's concept that white light incorporated all colors, but adhered to the Aristotelian view that color derived "from the primordial phenomenon of light and darkness, as affected or acted upon by semi-transparent mediums."[16]

Goethe recognized, however, that the eye sees only light and color and not objects themselves: "the eye sees in form, inasmuch as light, shade, and color together constitute that which to our vision distinguishes object from object."[17] Whereas Plato (see Chapter 12) argued that painted images could never express the true nature of an object, Goethe wrote that from "light, shade, and color, we construct the visible world, and thus, at the same time make painting possible, an art which the power of producing on a flat surface a much more perfect visible world than the actual one can be."[17]

Perhaps it was this philosophical concern, that reality derives from visual input, that led Goethe to distrust devices that distort the world, including optical aids and spectacles. He did not like visitors to wear glasses in his presence.[18] He could accept glasses on an old acquaintance with significant myopia, but he became furious with people who wore glasses as a fad or to a first meeting when they should have known better. Goethe himself was not myopic and did occasionally use an opera glass to see far away. In his novel *Wilhelm Meister,* the title character muses about the morality of optical technology, but in Pieter Strauss' words, "It is not the occasional use of a telescope, microscope or glasses by the highly cultivated individual that is felt to be dangerous here, but rather the wholesale, indiscriminate surrender to a fad that interposes a distorting lens between the world and that most important sense, the sense of sight."[18]

For all of its physical misinformation, Goethe's book on color is still a remarkable and careful document with respect to his psychophysical observations of how colors appear under specific experimental circumstances and how colors interact in our perceptual experience. Goethe was a good scientist in terms of documenting and recording the conditions of his observations, and his descriptions of afterimages, color contrast, shadows, and so on, are extraordinary. Toward the end of his life, he apparently came to regret his intemperant comments against Newton and was prepared to leave some of that material out of a new edition of his book.[19] Nevertheless, his book had considerable influence, perhaps in part because it was easier to read than the mathematical material written by physicists. He was a soul mate to Turner in his belief that light and dark were fundamentally more important than color. He wrote that "colors may be disposed rightly in themselves, but that a work may still appear motley, if they are falsely arranged in relation to light and shade."[20] He emphasized the fundamental antagonism, of yellow and blue:[21]

PLUS	MINUS
Yellow	Blue
Action	Negation
Light	Shadow
Brightness	Darkness
Force	Weakness
Warmth	Coldness
Proximity	Distance
Repulsion	Attraction
Affinity with acids	Affinity with alkalis

Turner added the words "light and shade" next to this list,[7] and in 1843 he painted a sequence of pictures that is of particular interest because Goethe is mentioned in one of the titles. The first painting (Fig. 8-4), *Shade and Darkness— The Evening of the Deluge,* is dominated by cool blues and grays and gives a sense of darkness and foreboding. The second (Fig. 8-5), titled *Light and Color (Goethe's Theory)—The Morning after the Deluge,* is dominated by brilliant yellow and light with frame of powerful red. It appears likely that the color and theme of these paintings derives from Goethe's list, although scholars have argued whether

FIGURE 8-4

Turner. *Shade and Darkness—The*
Evening of the Deluge.
Oil, 1843. (Clore Collection, Tate Gallery,
London/Art Resource, NY.)

The moon put forth her sign
of woe unheeded;/
But disobedience slept;
the dark'ning Deluge
closed around,/
And the last token came;
the giant framework floated,/
The roused beasts forsook their
nightly shelters screaming,/
And the beasts waded to the ark.

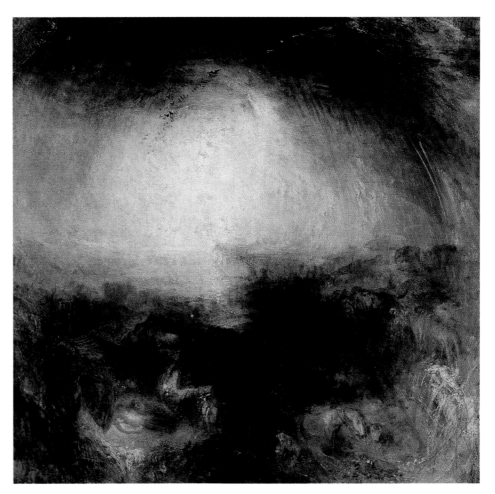

Turner was praising Goethe or criticizing him in these demonstrations.[22] While Turner approved of the dichotomy of light and shade, he differed from Goethe in believing that shadows and shade are a part of the spectrum of light and color rather than merely an absence of these qualities.

Many of Turner's sketchbooks include poetry as well as painting, but little of his poetry was ever published except as captions to his pictures. Although his paintings are grand and romantic, his poetry did not rise to similar heights.[23] The captions for his two paintings on the deluge are verses from a larger work called "Fallacies of Hope."

We have the luxury to look back, with the perspective of 150 years, on the interaction of three great minds: Newton, Goethe, and Turner. Newton's corpuscular theory of light has been modified by wave theory and quantum mechanics, but his brilliance in recognizing that white light is a composite of different wavelengths (i.e., different colors and different energies) remains a scientific landmark. Goethe's refusal to accept Newton's concept of light branded his own book as "nonscience," although it contained many rigorous and useful observations about color perception. There is renewed appreciation now for his skill as an observer and renewed awe at the abilities of this Renaissance man to understand so well both the scientific and ethereal aspects of human nature. Turner, caught between these philosophical giants, seemed both interested in science but skeptical of its value in art. He could accept Newton's physics and view color as a part of light, while also appreciating the emotional impact of light versus darkness in his artistic work.

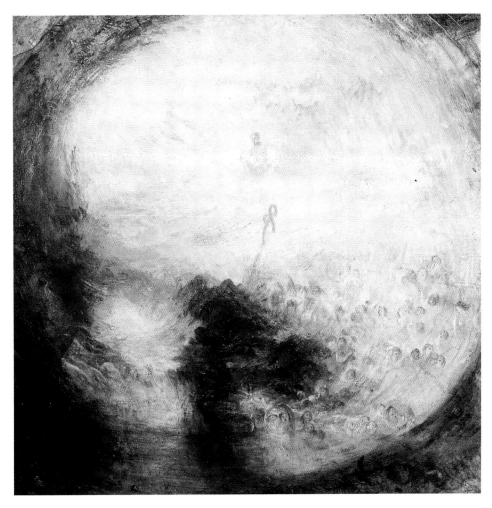

FIGURE   8-5

Turner. *Light and Color (Goethe's Theory)—The Morning after the Deluge.*

Oil, 1843. (Clore Collection, Tate Gallery, London/Art Resource, NY.)

The ark stook firm on Ararat; th' returning Sun/
Exhaled earth's humid bubbles, and emulous of light,/
Reflected her lost forms, each in prismatic guise/
Hope's harbinger, ephemeral as the summer fly/
Which rises, flits, expands, and dies.

There are perhaps some lessons in these musings. Artists have used scientific information variably in their work. Turner and Seurat read about theories of color but either misinterpreted them or relied on theories that are no longer valid. Yet their art is aesthetically magnificent. Modern artists such as M.C. Escher and Bridget Riley have expanded on images from science to create powerful and captivating images in their art. On the other hand, many great artists did not, to their knowledge, study science with respect to their art. To understand the nature of light, and the nature of vision, is to understand a part of the world, and it may explain why certain colors, contrasts, or shadows have a special visual impact on us. But this knowledge does not substitute for the sensitivity and innovation that separates the great artist from the illustrator. Turner and Seurat made choices in the construction of their paintings that were clearly affected by their interpretation of the science of the day; but the refinement and ultimate form of their paintings was determined by artistic rather than scientific judgment. We may not wish to go as far as Goethe and say that art is more perfect than the visible world, but we can surmise that it is a more perfect world because of art.

REFERENCES

1. Lindberg DC: *Theories of Vision from Al-Kindi to Kepler,* University of Chicago Press, Chicago, 1976.
2. Cantor G: *Anti-Newton.* In J Fauvel et al (eds): *Let Newton Be!* Oxford University Press, Oxford, 1988, pp. 203-221.
3. Magnus R: *Goethe as a Scientist,* Collier Books, New York, 1949 (translated by H. Norden).

4. Goethe W von: *Theory of Colours,* MIT Press, Cambridge, Mass., 1970 (translated by CL Eastlake reprint of 1840 edition; introduction by DB Judd).

5. Kohler K-H, Herr G, (eds): *Ludwig von Beethoven's Konversationhefte,* VEB Deutscher Verdag Fur Musik, Leipzig, 1972. Band I, Heft 9 (March 11-19, 1820), p. 348. Translated on the cover of Goethe.[4]

6. Gage J: *Color in Turner,* FA Praeger, New York, 1969, p. 110.

7. Gage J: Turner's annotated books: "Goethe's Theory of Colours," *Turner Studies* 4:34-52, 1984.

8. Whitley WT: *Art in England 1800-1820,* Macmillan, New York, 1928, pp. 179-180.

9. Whitley,[8] pp. 221-223.

10. Gage,[6] p. 210.

11. Whitley WT: *Art in England 1821-1834,* Cambridge University Press, Cambridge, Mass., 1930, pp. 132, 213.

12. Liebreich R: Turner and Mulready—On the effect of certain faults of vision on painting, with especial reference to their works, *Notices Proc Roy Inst* 6:450-463, 1872.

13. Cave K (ed): *The Diary of Joseph Farington,* vol. 3, Yale University Press, New Haven, Conn., 1979, p. 1075 (October 24, 1798); vol. 7, 1982, p. 2735 (April 26, 1806).

14. Trevor-Roper P: *The World through Blunted Sight,* rev ed, Penguin, London, 1988.

15. Goethe,[4] section 726, p. 287.

16. Goethe,[4] section 247, p. 102.

17. Goethe,[4] Introduction, pp. lii-liii.

18. Strauss DP: Why did Goethe hate glasses? *J Engl Germ Philol* 80:176-187, 1981.

19. Gage J: *Color and Culture,* Bulfinch Press, Boston, 1993, p. 202.

20. Goethe,[4] section 898, p. 344

21. Goethe,[4] section 696, p. 276.

22. Gage,[6] pp. 173-188; Gage,[19] pp. 201-204.

23. Gage J: *J.M.W. Turner "A Wonderful Range of Mind,"* Yale University Press, New Haven, Conn., 1987, pp. 181-205.

Chapter Nine

AN ARTIST WITH A COLOR VISION DEFECT

CHARLES MERYON

James G. Ravin and Philippe Lanthony

It is unusual for an important artist to have abnormal color vision. Artists who become aware of a defect in their color vision will usually stop working in color. They may utilize other media, such as sculpture or printmaking, which do not require normal color vision. Few individuals will enter art school if they are aware that their color perception is abnormal. One important figure in the history of art who had a congenital defect in his color vision, and who was aware of his abnormality, was the romantic etcher Charles Meryon (1821-1868) (Fig. 9-1). After studying art, Meryon realized that his abnormal color perception prevented him from being successful with oil paints. He then turned to printmaking. Some artists have acquired color vision defects, particularly in association with the development of cataracts, but this is quite different from a congenital defect.

> Meryon, even when he draws bricks, or granite or iron bars, or a railing of a bridge, puts into his etchings something of the human soul.
>
> —Vincent van Gogh[1]

VITA

Meryon was the illegitimate child of a Paris opera dancer and an English physician. His mother had an older child, a daughter, by an English nobleman. Charles' parents had a liaison in London, but a few months before his birth, his mother left England permanently. She detested England, calling it a "wretched country where it is always raining."[2] Charles' father acknowledged him as his son a few years later and allowed him to take the Meryon name. However, Dr. Meryon was

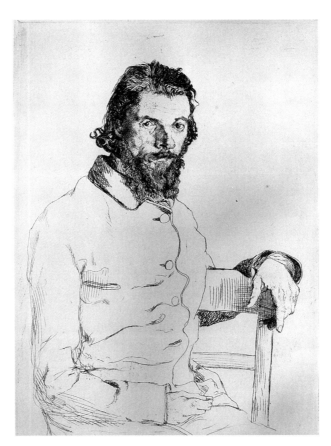

never able to provide Charles with the emotional support his son desired. This lack of paternal affection troubled Charles throughout his life. His mother had implored Dr. Meryon to recognize Charles legally, saying any "man who cannot name his father is very unhappy."[3] Dr. Meryon was constrained by the fact that he was married to an Englishwoman by whom he had two children. He did maintain a written correspondence with Charles' mother and with Charles and paid for his education. When he was 14, Charles met Dr. Meryon and his legitimate family in France and traveled with them for about a year. Charles and his father kept in touch via the mail for most of Charles' life. Charles' letters reveal his feelings about himself and his art, and they provide us with much that we know about his color perception.

Charles grew up in Paris with his mother and half sister. In a letter to Dr. Meryon, his mother described Charles' traits as an 8-year-old boy. "My Charles has a thousand good qualities, excessively sensitive, generous, sweet, spiritual, studious, diligent and somewhat unhappy. He hasn't the least self control. He is too young to have any strong feelings but his desires never end. If one cannot please him immediately he becomes most unhappy."[4] At age 14, Charles wrote his father, describing his desire to join the navy and his intention to illustrate the naval voyages he might undertake. Two years later, in 1837, he entered naval officers' school. His mother died the following year. His first voyage with the French navy was a Mediterranean cruise in 1840. On returning to France, he began formal art lessons. In 1842, at age 21, he embarked on a 4-year naval journey circumnavigating the globe, stopping in Brazil, New Zealand, Australia, and Tahiti. One of his goals during this voyage was to observe carefully and illustrate the exotic places he visited. He drew records of the natives and the landscape. Years later he utilized these drawings as source material for other works. He made

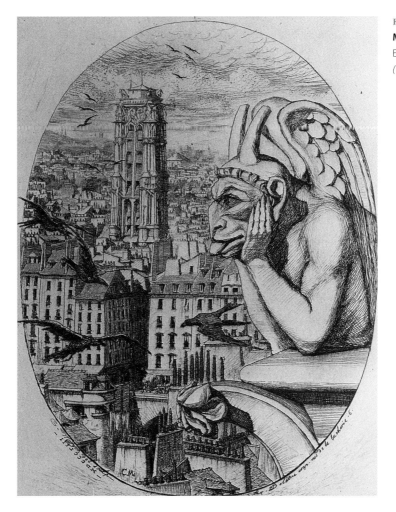

FIGURE   9-2
Meryon. *Le stryge.*
Etching, 1853.
(The Toledo Museum of Art.)

several lifelong friendships from this voyage. One of these close friends, Edouard Foley, later became a physician and aided him during periods of personal crisis.

A career as a military officer, in Meryon's opinion, was highly respectable. But at age 25 he wrote his father, describing his decision to leave the navy. "I have become tired of the profession which I have followed until now and I am still young enough to take up another. I am preparing to devote myself entirely to the study of art and to sacrifice everything I own to this end. I do not know what will happen to me. Perhaps I will become miserable, but I assure you that if I do not do this I will regret it for the rest of my life."[5]

This frank statement must be one of the clearest expositions of an artist's goals ever written. Meryon studied at the Louvre and with a pupil of the famous neo-classic artist Jacques-Louis David. His resignation from the navy became final in 1848. That same year he achieved official recognition when he exhibited a large scale drawing at the Salon, the annual state sponsored exhibition.

However, Meryon was never able to translate his drawing into an oil painting. He realized that his congenital color vision defect made work in oils too difficult. Although no journalists seemed to have noticed his drawing at the Salon, the composition caught the attention of an etcher, Eugène Bléry. The two artists met, lived, and worked together for about 2 years. In 1849 Meryon began work on his most famous series of etchings, the *Eaux-fortes sur Paris* (Scenes of Old Paris) (Figs. 9-2 and 9-3), the medieval city that Napoleon III and Baron Haussmann demolished during the Second Empire (1851-1870).

FIGURE 9-3
Meryon. *Le petit pont.*
Etching. *(The Toledo Museum of Art.)*

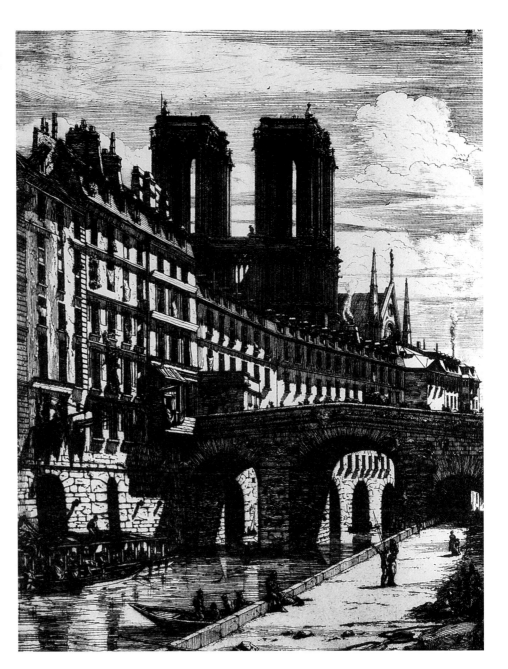

THE COLOR DEFECT

Meryon's abnormal color vision apparently was not discovered when he entered the navy. Color testing was not part of the admission process at that time. During his early art studies, in the 1840s, he began with sepia and then moved to the medium of watercolor. In 1841 he wrote his father that "I have stopped use of sepia, to begin watercolor, which naturally offers so many more possibilities."[6] He soon realized his color vision was defective. He wrote his father that he hoped to overcome this obstacle through practice. In 1846, only a few weeks after devoting himself to art, he faced the color problem directly. "This color defect of which I speak is such that I often prefer beautiful black prints, in which one can see the graduation of shading, to the more vivid effects of painting."[7] Despite this admission, Meryon did not give up painting immediately. He wrote his friend, the

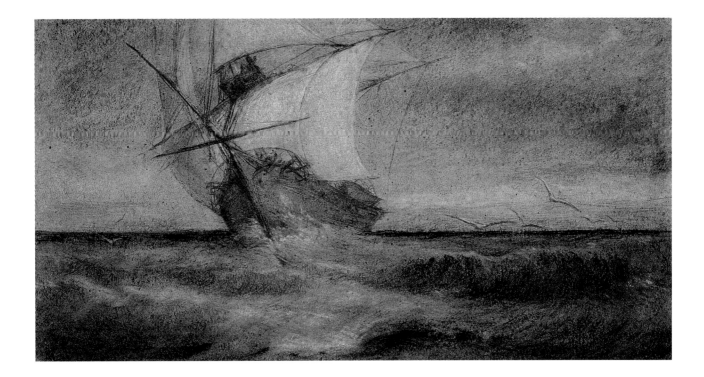

medical student Foley, that he intended to continue his plan to paint noble themes. He drew up plans for future subjects. One was Joan of Arc surrounded by her executioners. Others included whaling subjects and themes he had encountered during his voyage to the South Seas. For many of the compositions, Meryon envisioned evening light. The dramatic possibilities of oblique lighting with strong contrasts of light and shade planned for oils became important features of his later etchings.

Very few of Meryon's works in color have survived. A lone work in oil is known only from a photograph in the Bibliothèque Nationale in Paris. A pastel entitled *Ghost Ship* (Fig. 9-4) is in the collection of the Louvre.[8,9] Undoubtedly he created this from memory after becoming aware of his color vision defect. It is interesting to note that in this pastel Meryon avoided the colors that give color-deficient artists difficulty, red and green. To understand this, we need to understand the differences in colors seen by normal individuals and color-deficient individuals.

As discussed in Chapter 1, hereditary color deficiency generally results from an absence or abnormality of the gene for the red- or green-catching pigment in the retina. The genes for red and green color sensitivity are on the X (sex) chromosome, and color blindness is almost exclusively a disorder of males. Severely color-deficient individuals lack either the perception of green or red, so every color at the warm end of the spectrum looks the same (and is most often called yellow subjectively).

If a painter with normal color vision places on his palette the principal colors of the spectrum, he can do so in a circle of colors with red at 12:00, purple and cold colors from 12:00 to 6:00, and warm tones from 6:00 to 12:00 (Fig. 9-5). The colors opposite each other in this circle are complementary tones. Red at 12:00 is, for example, complementary to blue-green at 6:00. There is no uncolored area, either white or gray, in this color circle.

If an artist with a severe red-green color vision defect looks at this palette, he sees it differently from the normal individual. The palette appears to him essen-

FIGURE   9-5
Normal color spectrum.

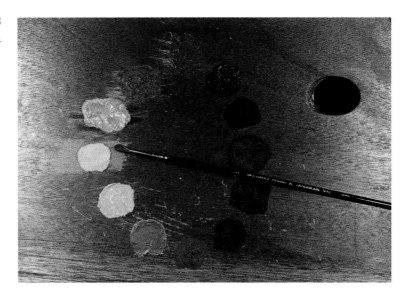

FIGURE   9-6
Color-deficient spectrum.

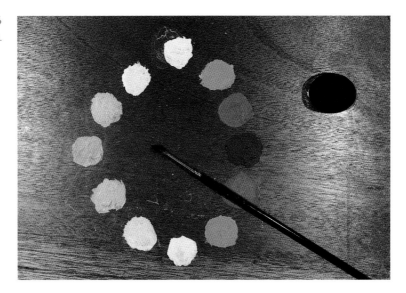

tially comprising two colors. Blue is within the cold colors from 12:00 to 6:00, and yellow (or his sensation for the warm colors) is located on the warm side from 6:00 to 12:00 (Fig. 9-6). Between these two pigments, the color-deficient artist sees a relatively uncolored zone, white or grayish. To him, a balance between warm and cold colors is equivalent to a mixture of *all* colors, that is, white. The result is that the color-deficient artist who desires to reproduce a blue-green tint (i.e., a color that falls in the gray zone between warm and cold colors) hesitates in choosing between a purplish red, a gray, and a blue-green, all of which appear to be nearly the same to him. He has one chance in three to be correct. In the same fashion, outside of the gray or uncolored zone, he will confuse yellow, green, and orange, and he may confuse blue and purple. It would require a bit of luck for the color-deficient artist to chose a color that appears the same to a normal individual.[10] Meryon's choices of colors in the phantom ship reveal the color deficient artist's characteristic division of the world into blue and yellow. The sky has an unusual cast to it, being overly yellow-orange, and the sea is overly blue, lacking the normal green component.

Despite his color vision defect, Meryon was able to depict contrasts in light and dark. Certainly his choice of the medium of etching stresses the nuances of contrasts. In some of his prints Meryon used two inks, red and black. Although we do not completely understand how Meryon perceived red, he must have seen it as lighter than black. Meryon did not own a press and had to take his plates to printers. His prints appear on a variety of papers—fine light cream laid paper, white paper, thicker beige-colored paper, and green paper. Again, we are not certain how Meryon perceived the tones of these papers. He may have perceived few differences and may have been influenced by other individuals in the selection of the papers. We can assume that he would have appreciated the textural differences between various papers.

Utilizing stark contrasts of black and white with little gradation of tone, Meryon created a chillingly eerie atmosphere. This is particularly effective in his etchings of the medieval aspects of Paris. These prints were admired by the poet Charles-Pierre Baudelaire and the writer Victor Hugo. Hugo wrote Baudelaire "Since you know Meryon, tell him that his splendid etchings, with nothing but shadow and brightness, light and dark, have dazzled me."[11]

A SAD ENDING

Vincent van Gogh, one of the great colorists of all time, was well aware of Meryon's work in black and white. Like van Gogh, Meryon came to a tragic end. Both of these artistic geniuses developed a mental illness that overcame them. In 1868 Meryon was admitted to the asylum of Charenton, where he died. Paul Gachet, M.D., best known for his relationship with van Gogh, visited Meryon and sketched several portraits of him at the asylum. The admitting diagnosis was "lypemania," now an obsolete term denoting a form of depression. Hints of this were present during his year in the navy, in terms of long-lasting periods of ennui and inaction. Later he developed hallucinations and feelings of persecution. His oral intake was very poor, and he died in an unfortunate state, at the age of 47. He is survived by his brilliant creations.

— **REFERENCES** —

1. van Gogh V: *The Complete Letters of Vincent van Gogh,* New York Graphic Society, Greenwich, Conn., 1959, Letter 136.
2. Fama PG: Charles Meryon: A biographical and psychiatric reassessment, *N Z Med J* 78:448-455, 1973.
3. Chaspoux N: Letter dated March 30, 1823, British Museum. In J Ducros: *Charles Meryon*, Musée de la Marine, Paris, 1968, Number 287.
4. Chaspoux N: Letter dated July 1829, British Museum. In Ducros,[3] Number 297.
5. Meryon C: Letter, British Museum. In Ducros,[3] Number 366.
6. Drost WWR: Documents nouveaux sur l'oeuvre et la vie de Charles Meryon, *Gazette des beaux-arts* 63:230, 1964.
7. Meryon C: Letter, British Museum. In Ducros,[3] Number 367.
8. Collins R: The landscape and historical paintings of Charles Meryon, *Turnbull Library Record* 8:4-16, 1975.
9. Meryon C: Letter, British Museum. In Ducros,[3] Number 781.
10. Lanthony P: Dyschromatopsies et art pictural, *J Fr Opthalmol* 14:510-519, 1991.
11. Meryon C: Letter, British Museum. In Ducros,[3] Number 449.

Chapter Ten

THE VISION OF VINCENT VAN GOGH

James G. Ravin and Michael F. Marmor

Vincent van Gogh (1853-1890) painted in a unique and appealing style. His life, full of tragedy, has captured the public's interest. No other artist has ever had a painting sell at public auction for as much money as this man did. Sadly, he struggled to sell his works during his lifetime and succeeded only rarely. His medical problems have led to a very long list of possible diagnoses. A strong case has been made for psychiatric entities, with manic depressive (bipolar) illness frequently mentioned to explain the episode of his ear and his ultimate suicide.[1,2] Epilepsy was entertained as a diagnosis on his admission to the hospital in Arles and the asylum at St. Remy during the last 2 years of his life.[3] Infectious diseases and toxins have also been considered as diagnoses or adjunctive factors. Recently, a metabolic disease, acute intermittent porphyria, has been proposed as an all inclusive diagnosis.[4] This disorder can have protean neurological manifestations, including pain and mental disturbance, and is believed to account for the madness of King George III of England.[5] Van Gogh's family history is suggestive of a hereditary disease (brother Theo and sister Wilhelmina had related symptoms and insanity). However, there is no direct evidence of acute intermittent porphyria in van Gogh (such as a letter describing the characteristic dark urine), and his personality disturbance was rather persistent and prominent over many years.

VINCENT'S EYESIGHT

Considering the artist's unusual approach to art, some critics have wondered if his eyesight was normal. Furthermore, some of his putative physical disorders such as toxic exposures and acute intermittent porphyria can affect vision. The only medical data are a vision examination by his last personal physician, the well-known Dr. Paul Ferdinand Gachet.[6] Van Gogh's vision was tested by Gachet in May 1890 at Gachet's country home at Auvers, not at his office in Paris. Vincent's younger brother, Theo, had brought Gachet up to date about Vincent's health status. The examination was informal, and in no sense a complete one, to avoid creating any sense of anxiety on Vincent's part. Gachet was a physician for one of the French railroad companies and was called on at times to test the vision of workers. He had a visual acuity chart on the wall, next to a painting by Pissarro. The chart piqued Vincent's curiosity, and he asked Gachet about it. The doctor tested the artist's vision and found it excellent. He needed no glasses for reading or for distance. When tested with the color vision materials used for the railroad personnel, again the results were perfectly normal. This is the extent of the data available on testing Vincent's eyes during his last year of life.

HALOES OF COLORS

Colored haloes around sources of light are found in several of Vincent's most famous paintings, including *Starry Night* and *The Night Cafe* (Fig. 10-1). Certainly van Gogh was not the first artist to paint curvilinear forms of color around light sources. This technique had been employed previously, for symbolic reasons in religious paintings and to create a sense of atmosphere in landscapes. Nevertheless, this visual phenomenon has given rise to the idea that van Gogh may have suffered from a form of glaucoma, since this disease can cause colored haloes to surround lights.[7] Colored haloes are caused by diffraction of light, the breaking up of white light into its component parts, the color spectrum. Anyone who wears glasses or contact lenses for distant vision has noticed that if the lenses are filmy, in the presence of fog or at night, colored haloes can appear around streetlights or automobile headlights. But Vincent did not wear glasses. The cornea itself can diffract light if it becomes abnormally swollen (edematous), and angle closure glaucoma is one of the few diseases capable of causing such swelling intermittently. In this form of glaucoma, a marked elevation of intraocular pressure overcomes the cornea's ability to pump fluid out. However, there is no evidence from van Gogh's lifetime that he ever suffered from glaucoma. In his letters there is no mention of the characteristic symptoms of this disease—eye pain, nausea, and sudden loss of vision. Furthermore, acute angle closure glaucoma is very rarely found in patients under age 40, and Vincent died at age 37. In short, there are many reasons to discount this diagnosis, and glaucoma is hardly necessary to explain an artistic device used by so many artists over the ages.

YELLOW VISION

A yellow coloration dominates many of van Gogh's paintings.[8] This is particularly evident in his late works. (It may seem a bit strange to discuss a late phase of an artist who lived to be only 37.) Examples of works with a marked yellow cast include *The Night Cafe* (see Fig. 10-1), his wheat fields, and the house at Arles

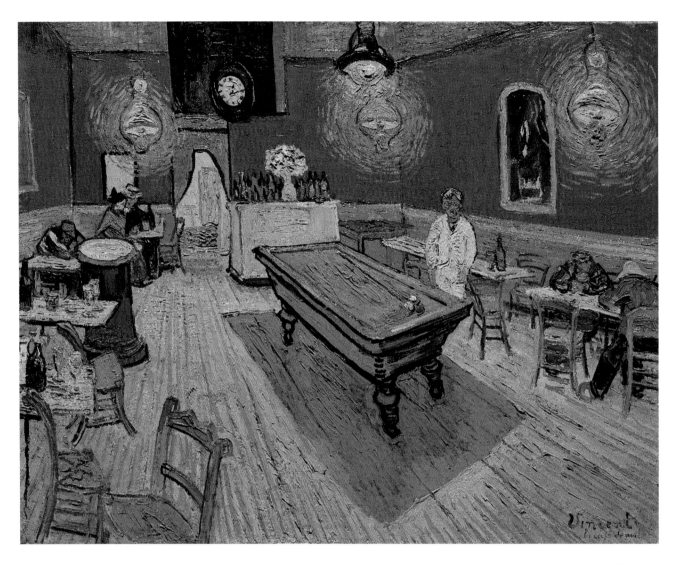

FIGURE 10-1

van Gogh. *The Night Cafe
(Le Café de Nuit).*

(Yale University Art Gallery.)

simply entitled *The Yellow House*. A yellowishness characterizes Vincent's flesh in many of the self-portraits (Fig. 10-2), particularly the late ones, even though he is not known to have been jaundiced.

DIGITALIS

After Vincent cut off part of his left ear in late December 1888, he was admitted to the hospital in Arles. He was under the care of Felix Rey, a 23-year-old intern who had graduated from the University of Montpellier medical school. That school was an ancient one, and the level of education there in psychiatry was excellent. Rey believed that Vincent was suffering from a form of epilepsy. Rey's friend Aussoleil, a classmate at the University of Montpellier, was an intern at a psychiatric hospital nearby. Aussoleil wrote his thesis for the medical degree on the subject of epilepsy, and he may have influenced Rey in making the diagnosis of a seizure disorder for Vincent.[3]

Treatment of seizure disorders at that time often included the use of digitalis. Digitalis was one of the medications for which there was a large body of pharmacologic knowledge. Although its main use was in cardiology, it was also used for many other purposes. Dr. Paul Gachet, Vincent's last physician, was well aware of this drug, and of the importance of proper dosage in its use.

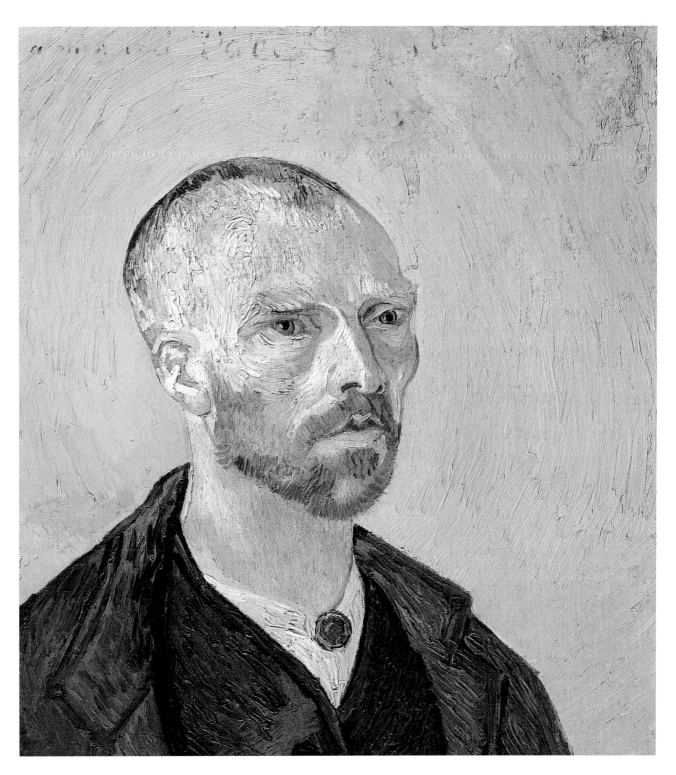

Vincent painted portraits of only two of his many physicians, Drs. Rey and Gachet (Fig. 10-3). He painted Rey one time and Gachet twice. The extremely famous painting of Gachet, auctioned by Christie's in 1990, is the most expensive painting ever to have been sold at a public auction. It went to a Japanese businessman for the astronomical sum of $82.5 million. In the foreground of his painting, and also in the version illustrated here, is a sprig of purple foxglove plant, from which digitalis is derived. Vincent had wanted to include something

FIGURE   10-2

van Gogh. *Self-Portrait (dedicated to Paul Gauguin).*

Oil on Canvas, 1888. *(Courtesy of the Fogg Art Museum, Harvard University Art Museums. Bequest of Collection of Maurice Wertheim, Class of 1906.)*

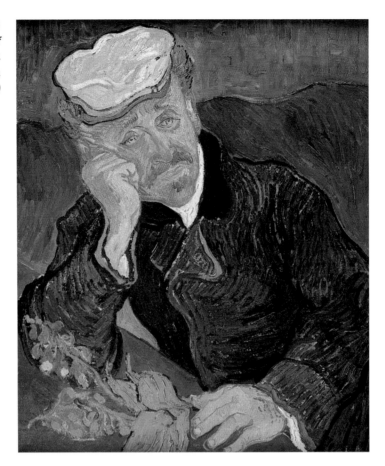

in the painting that would indicate the subject was a physician and Gachet suggested the foxglove, symbolic of his interest in diseases of the heart.[9] Although there is no evidence that Vincent was ever treated with digitalis for the diagnosis of a seizure disorder, or for any other diagnosis, the question has frequently arisen because yellow vision can be a symptom of digitalis toxicity.

Gachet has been accused of mismanaging van Gogh's care, by giving him an excessive dose of digitalis.[10] However, there are several reasons for believing that Gachet could not have possibly treated him with a dose sufficient to cause ocular side effects. First, Gachet was well aware of the potential for problems with this medication. He even wrote that digitalis could be deadly. In his unpublished treatise on military ophthalmia, Gachet states, "We understand the physiologic effects of this plant well enough today to be afraid of its dangers, and strongly advise against its use, since it can produce syncope by slowing the heartbeat and it can cause paralysis of that organ."[11]

Second, although digitalis was a medication on the homeopathic medical formulary at the time Gachet was practicing medicine, he could never have given this drug in a dose sufficiently high to cause toxicity. The 1835 version of Hahnemann's homeopathic formulary lists 73 indications for treatment with digitalis. The list includes melancholic thoughts, hypochondria, mental illness, headache, nausea, vomiting, pain in the eyes, swelling of the eyelids, tearing, and inflammation of the eyes.[12] However, homeopathic doses are so extremely low, minute fractions of allopathic doses, that toxicity is not possible. Although educated in traditional allopathic medicine, Gachet followed homeopathic formulas when it came to therapy. Camille Pissarro had recommended to Theo van Gogh that Gachet be engaged as Vincent's physician. Pissarro knew Gachet would treat

Vincent sympathetically and he knew that the doctor was an advocate of home-opathy. Gachet had even treated Pissarro's mother.

Third, Gachet was not convinced that van Gogh suffered from a seizure disorder, the working diagnosis made when Vincent was admitted to the hospital in Arles and continued during his confinement at the asylum in St. Remy. Gachet's son described the scenario in May 1890 when Vincent arrived in Auvers. Prior to that time, the two had never met, although Gachet was familiar with van Gogh's work. He had seen Vincent's paintings at the exhibitions of the Independents in 1888, 1890, and 1899. From his conversations with Theo, Gachet was optimistic that he could be of help. As soon as he met Vincent face to face, however, he realized that medications would be impossible with him and that the diagnosis must be changed from "crises nerveuses epileptoides" to "maladie mentale circulaire."[13] This latter diagnosis represents an earlier wording for what is known today as manic-depressive (bipolar) illness.

The concept that manic-depressive illness is a single disease entity was first described during the middle of the nineteenth century in France.[14] Jean Pierre Falret (1794-1870), a psychiatrist who worked at the Salpêtrière in Paris, described an abnormality in which moods swinging from mania to melancholy and back are separated by intervals of perfect lucidity. He described the states of excitation and depression, the hallucinations, the hereditary aspects of the disease, and the need to vary the medication used to treat the disease.[15] Toward the end of the nineteenth century the term "manic-depressive illness" was introduced, and in the twentieth century the word "bipolar" came into use. Gachet studied at the Salpêtrière as an extern on Falret's service in 1855. In 1858 Gachet published his thesis for the medical degree on the subject of melancholy,[16] and he retained an intense interest in mental illness throughout his medical career.

SANTONIN

Santonin is another medication that can acutely cause yellow vision. It has been available as an antimicrobial agent against gastrointestinal worms for nearly 2 centuries. Arnold and Loftus have suggested that Vincent may have taken santonin.[8] It was recommended a century ago as a preventive medication and utilized for rather imprecise indications. Vincent was interested in health questions and owned a copy of Dr. François-Vincent Raspail's popular *Manuel Annuaire de la Santé*,[17] which he portrayed in his painting *Still Life: Drawing Board with Onions* of 1889. Raspail recommended the use of santonin for gastrointestinal disorders, and Vincent had some digestive problems. Arnold and Loftus also feel that van Gogh suffered from pica (abnormal craving) for chemicals similar to santonin, including camphor, thujone, and turpentine.[8] This pica could have induced him to take santonin. He did use large doses of camphor to fight off insomnia. He frequently drank absinthe, which contains thujone as an active ingredient. The artist Signac reported that Vincent wanted to drink a large volume of turpentine while he was with him.

NONMEDICAL FACTORS

Do van Gogh's canvases support a diagnosis of xanthopsia (yellow vision)? To do so, a significant number of paintings should show a dominance of yellow tints with no white, blue, or violet surface.[18,19] Some canvases come close to this, the most interesting being *The Night Cafe* (see Fig. 10-1). Nevertheless, these examples are rare in his work, and are intermixed among paintings extending back to Holland (Fig. 10-4). What is more striking is that the importance of yellow is most often balanced by an abundance of blues. Vincent insisted on a balance between

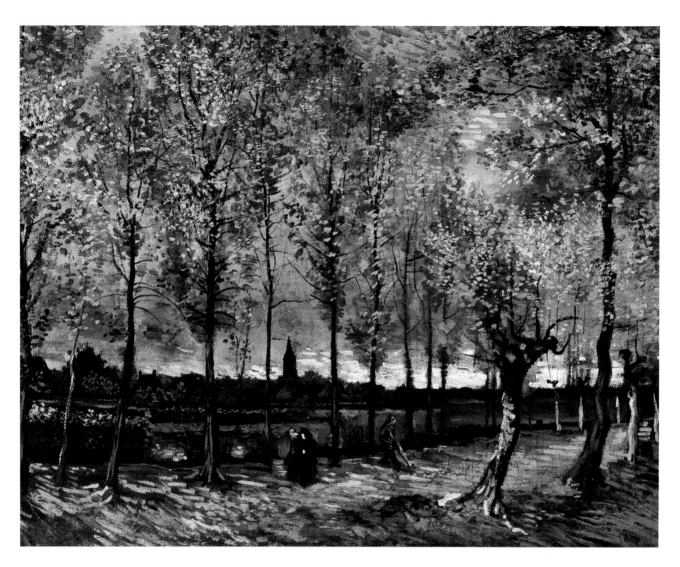

FIGURE 10-4

van Gogh. *Poplar Avenue Near Nuenen.*

(Museum Boymans-van Beuningen, Rotterdam.)

yellow and blue in his correspondence, and this may be found in a number of his paintings. Since there is no evidence that he ever took digitalis and only a possibility that he used santonin, at best one can say that he might have had some memories of medication-induced episodes with yellow vision. The greatest caution should be taken in interpreting the eyesight of artists based on their works. Van Gogh is certainly not the first artist whose predominant use of yellow has been attributed to an ocular problem. Others include Reni, Signorelli, Verrio, El Greco, Titian, and Turner (see Chapter 8), although the evidence is marginal that ocular disease (such as a yellowish cataract) was responsible in any of these cases. There are only a few artists, such as Monet (see Chapter 14), for whom alterations in color usage and color vision has been satisfactorily documented as due to disease. Medical historiography has at times been too eager to fit unusual diseases to symptoms, perhaps as an outgrowth of our medical education system, which trains young doctors to think more of possibilities (lest a diagnosis be missed) than probabilities.[20]

Many nonmedical explanations can account for van Gogh's use of yellow. First, he had an intellectual fascination with color throughout his career, and his letters are filled with discourses about the importance and use of colors. He was constantly experimenting with different tonalities. Like many artists (see Chapters 8 and 11), van Gogh studied the color science of his day and tried at times to fol-

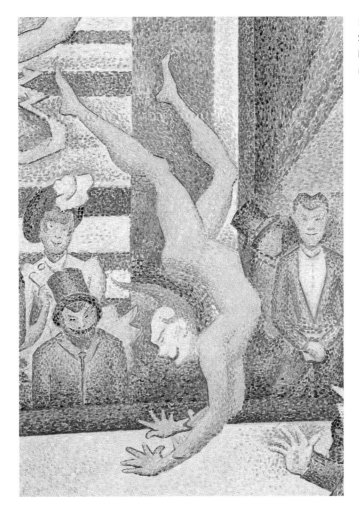

FIGURE   11-1
Seurat. *Le cirque.*
Detail. Oil on canvas, 1890-91.
(© Photo R.M.N. Musée d'Orsay, Paris.)

The phenomenon of optical mixture has been known since antiquity. It was described in Ptolemy's *Optics* in its two forms, rotating disks and colored spots.[2] It was used in the making of carpets, mosaics, and textiles. And when a critic claimed that the Neo-Impressionist painters were "too scientific," Signac replied, "The lowest Oriental weaver knows as much about this as they do."[3]

—— VISUAL TEXTURE ——

The texture of a surface is the quality of being simultaneously uniform and heterogeneous, due to the repetitive distribution of elementary units. In painting, three kinds of physical textures should be described: the physical texture of the object being used as a model; the physical texture of the surface on which the painting is made (e.g., wood, stone, paper, canvas, etc.); and the physical texture of the painted image, which is made of points, lines, dots, spots, brush strokes, and so on.

The texture perceived visually by the beholder is the result of the combination of these three physical textures. In classical painting the main purpose of an artist was the exact reproduction of the texture of the objects used as model, and good technique tried to mask texture of the canvas or wood base and of the painted image. There are many examples of this in Flemish and Dutch painting and also, by the way, in modern American photo-realism. In Seurat's technique, however, the painted texture of dots is very apparent even at casual examination, for the main purpose of the painter is not the reproduction of object texture but rather the production of a luminous and colored effect. The historical contribution of Seurat was to clearly understand that the texture made of discrete colored units could be used in a systematic way to obtain an optical mixture. Seurat's conception was the result of a long and meditative evolution,[4] which did not culminate before 1886. The best illustrations of the technique are found in *Les Poseuses, La Parade, Le Cirque* (Fig. 11-1), and in his marine landscapes.

OPTICAL MIXTURE IN POINTILLISM

— COLORIMETRIC STUDY —

To study optical mixture, I have used the method of rotating disks. Bicolored disks were placed on a rotor and spun to induce an optical mixture of the two colors. The advantage of this technique is that it allows one to isolate the three psychophysiological attributes of color, that is, hue, saturation, and lightness (Fig. 11-2). The hues of the optical mixture were, generally speaking, intermediate between the hues of the two components. The saturation of the mixture was generally lower than the respective saturations of the two components. The minimum saturation occurred with complimentary colors in which the resulting mixture looked gray (this tendency to gray was an important feature of optical mixture). Finally, the lightness of the mixture was intermediate between the lightness of the components. In general, the mixtures looked rather light, as shown in Fig. 11-2. This demonstrates the main difference between optical and subtractive mixtures: an optical mixture gives rise to a much greater lightness than a subtractive mixture made of the two same components. This point was strongly emphasized by the Neo-Impressionists.

— COMPOSITION OF SEURAT'S PALETTE —

Seurat's palette is shown in Fig. 11-3 (see Minervino).[5] The first row of 11 pure hues (i.e., colors directly out of the tubes) has neither black nor dark colors such as brown. The single subtractive mixture of hues the painter allowed himself was between two contiguous hues—"as in the spectrum," said Signac.[3] Thus, Seurat had

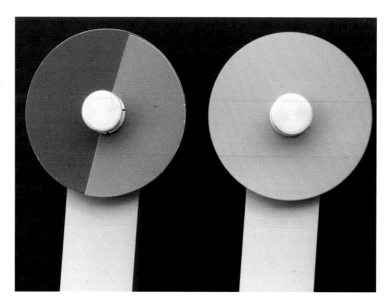

FIGURE 11-2
Optical mixture produced by rotating disk. *Left:* The two halves of the disk are different in hue, saturation, and lightness. *Right:* Rapid rotation of the disk gives rise to an optical mixture of which the hue is intermediate between red and green, the saturation is low, and the lightness is high, to a much greater degree than an equivalent subtractive mixture.

22 hues available, as in the color circle of Rood, whose book he had certainly read.[6] Seurat never used subtractive mixtures of distant hues on the palette, but he did make mixtures of each hue with the white pigment in the second row of the palette, thus producing an intermediate row between the saturated hues and the pure whites.

It is important to emphasize that the 11 basic hues of Seurat (or, better, the 22 hues, when he mixed adjacent colors) suitably overlaid the whole spectrum. The oft-mentioned analogy between Seurat's technique and a television screen is not exact. On a television screen all the hues are obtained by an additive mixture of only three basic hues: blue, green, and red, corresponding to the three types of cone photoreceptors in the retina (trichromatic principle) (see Chapter 1). But Seurat did not need to make a trichromatic synthesis, since he had at his disposal 11 (or 22) hues and could use them directly, putting them on canvas in little spots which he allowed to dry to avoid subtractive mixtures. The optical mixture of Seurat was in no way intended as a mixture of just three fundamental primaries.

THE UTILITY OF OPTICAL MIXTURE

If Seurat didn't use optical mixture on the basis of trichromatic theory, of what use was it in his paintings? Some experiments with rotating disks provide the answer. Reproductions of Seurat's paintings were cut in a circular shape and mounted on the rotor (Fig. 11-4). These images can be analyzed with respect to hue, saturation and lightness. Seurat often used not only two, but three, four, and even five different *hues* in juxtaposition, leaving the eye the task of optical mixture. The method of rotating disks shows that the results were often unexpected with subtle combinations of hues giving rise to delicate shades and color modulations. The optical mixture lowered the *saturation;* even quite pure and saturated colors, when mixed in this fashion, result in rather faint colors. The optical mixtures were, on the whole, rather *light.* Compare the motionless disks in the left column of Fig. 11-4 with the rotated disks in the right column. These experiments demonstrate that Seurat's optical mixture of colored spots resulted in an overall attenuation of the attributes of color. This was in direct accord with the aesthetic principle of Seurat that art is harmony. He sought a soft modulation of the hues and saturation, and general lightness, to obtain gentle effects, concordance without discordance, and transitions without contrast between the colored dots. An example of this is given in Fig. 11-5.

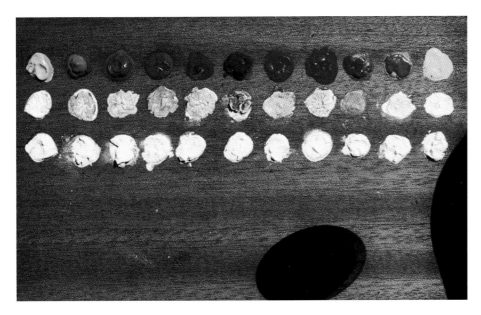

FIGURE **11-3**

Seurat's palette. It included three rows of pigments: a first row made of 11 pure hues, beginning with green-yellow, and aligned according to the order of the spectrum; a second row made of 11 white pigment spots; and a third row, between the other two, made of individual mixtures of each pure hue with the corresponding white.

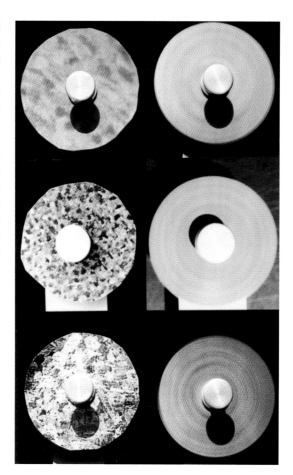

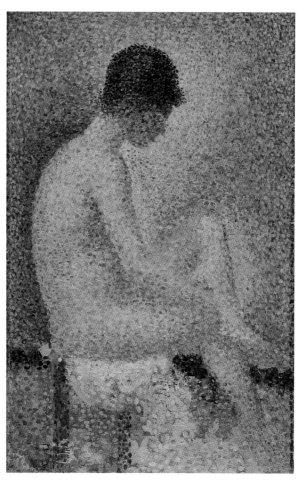

LIMITS OF THE OPTICAL MIXTURE

The experiments with rotating disks also demonstrate another important fact. Each of the colors obtained on the rotating disks of Fig. 11-4 could also have been obtained by a suitable subtractive mixture, but different pigments would have been required. In other words, the optical mixture is not necessary as a method for obtaining Seurat's choice of colors. What was, then, the reason for his rather complicated and time-consuming technique? The answer is that optical mixture is only half of the story. Spatial features (i.e., texture) are equally important to Seurat's method of painting.

VISUAL TEXTURE IN POINTILLISM

The viewer who looks at Seurat's painting close up perceives a surface made of little colored spots, distributed in a fairly monotonous manner on the canvas, that gives the impression of a regular grain. Of course, this regularity is only relative; Seurat's pixels are rather rough in comparison with those on a television screen (Fig. 11-6). Nevertheless, the density of the colored dots and their overall equality of size determines the pictorial texture of the painting, and one can see the visual effect of their spacing and contrast.

RELATIONSHIP BETWEEN CONTRAST SENSITIVITY AND OPTICAL MIXTURE

Contrast sensitivity is the capacity of the eye to discriminate two juxtaposed stimuli according to differences (i.e., contrast) in hue, saturation, or lightness. Optical mixture can be considered the reverse of contrast sensitivity, as it diminishes the viewer's capacity to discriminate between juxtaposed stimuli. Contrast sensitivity is usually studied by means of grids or gratings of various spatial fre-

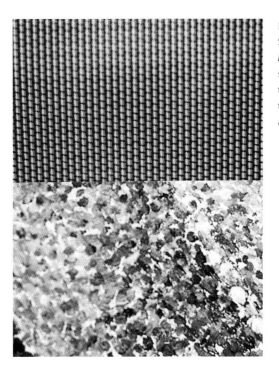

FIGURE 11-6
Seurat's pixels. *Top:* Television screen. *Bottom:* Seurat's painting. The television screen is perfectly regular and the pixels are small. Nevertheless, the two surfaces give a similar appearance of colored visual texture.

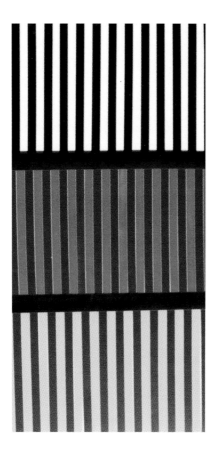

quencies (i.e., fineness of spacing). There are three forms of contrast sensitivity with respect to pointillism: (1) achromatic contrast sensitivity, that is, a contrast of lightness alone, studied by means of a unicolored grating, usually black and white (Fig. 11-7, top); (2) chromatic contrast sensitivity, or a contrast in hue alone, studied by means of a bicolored grating in which the colors have the same lightness (see Fig. 11-7, middle); and (3) contrast sensitivity with gratings that vary simultaneously in hue and lightness, as in bicolored and biluminous grating (see Fig. 11-7, bottom).

Experiments have shown that contrast sensitivity is optimal at a certain spatial frequency. There is also a maximum, or threshold, spatial frequency beyond which an observer is unable to discriminate the components of a grating. In other words, above the threshold, the eye only recognizes optical mixture. The important point, shown in Fig. 11-8, is that these thresholds are very different for achromatic and for chromatic sensitivity (see, e.g., Mullen).[7] The threshold for achromatic sensitivity occurs at a higher spatial frequency (30 to 40 cycles/degree), that is, it extends to finer lines or smaller dots, than the threshold for chromatic sensitivity (10 to 15 cycles/degree). Thus, there is a range of dissociation between the two thresholds of optical mixture.

When an observer looks at a grating that varies simultaneously in hue and lightness (as in Fig. 11-7, bottom), its visual appearance is related to spatial frequency in the following ways: at low spatial frequency (e.g., below 10 cycles/degree), one perceives a biluminous and bicolored grating (in the example of Fig. 11-7, dark red and light yellow); at high spatial frequency (e.g., beyond 40 cycles/degree), one no longer perceives the grating but instead only a uniformly colored and luminous surface (in this example some orange) by means of perfect optical mixture. But at intermediate spatial frequency (e.g., between 10 and 40

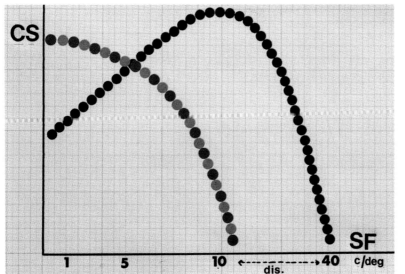

FIGURE 11-8

Achromatic and chromatic contrast sensitivity curves. *Abcissa:* Spatial frequency (c/degree = cycles/degree). *Ordinate:* Contrast sensitivity. *Black circles:* Achromatic contrast sensitivity. *Colored circles:* Chromatic contrast sensitivity. The maximal spatial frequency that can be resolved is different for achromatic and chromatic contrast; this leaves a dissociation (dis.) between the two thresholds of optical mixture.

FIGURE 11-9

Von Bezold assimilation. The same red color near yellow looks somewhat orange, and near blue looks somewhat purple. This is in contradiction to the law of color contrast.

cycles/degree), one is in the range of dissociation between achromatic and chromatic contrast sensitivity, and the surface appears uniform in hue but varying in lightness (in this example, a grating of light and dark orange). These effects can be demonstrated by changing the distance at which these gratings are viewed. In practice, this oversimplified description is complicated by some other visual effects. The most important is the von Bezold assimilation phenomenon, which is at odds with the law of simultaneous contrast. According to the latter, as enunciated by Chevreul,[8] when the eye sees two contiguous colors, they will appear as dissimilar as possible both in hue and lightness. Von Bezold observed that the reverse phenomenon can occur, under certain circumstances, when color patterns become fine, interlaced, or both (an example is given in Fig. 11-9). According to the careful analysis of Helson,[9] the von Bezold phenomenon can be considered a first step toward optical mixture, and it helps to produce a smooth visual continuum from simultaneous contrast to complete optical mixture.

— SPATIAL FREQUENCY IN SEURAT'S PAINTING —

Although the spatial frequency of the colored dots on the surface of Seurat's canvas is relatively constant, an observer can vary the spatial frequency simply by changing the viewing distance. Several situations are possible. When one is close to the canvas, the spatial frequency of the dots is low, and one perceives a textured surface made of spots, a grain with various hues, saturations, and lightness; these spots appear in vivid colors, and the whole painting gives the impression of a multicolored area. But Seurat's paintings were not intended for such close examination, any more than a television screen is made to be seen at, say, a distance of 10 centimeters.

Conversely, when one is a long distance from the canvas, the spatial frequency of the dots is high. One no longer sees colored spots but only large surfaces of rather uniform color with some shaded gradations. This is the range of spatial frequency in which optical mixture is complete.

When one views a Seurat painting at some mean distance between these two extremes, however, the perceived spatial frequency of the dots is in the range of dissociation in which optical mixture is possible for hue but not for lightness. This makes the appearance of the painting somewhat peculiar: one sees a surface approximately uniform in hue but on which there are a lot of little dark dots. It is precisely this aspect of grain that had struck the first beholders of these paintings and from which is born the term "pointillism" (Fig. 11-10).

FIGURE 11-10

Seurat. *Poseuse de Dos.*

Oil on Wood, 1886-1887. *(© Photo R.M.N. Musée d'Orsay, Paris.)*

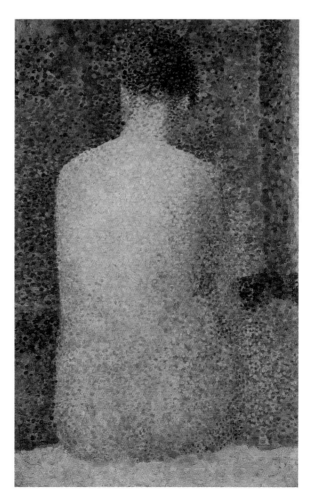

MODULATIONS OF SEURAT'S PAINTING
BY VISUAL TEXTURE

Up to this point, I have described Seurat's paintings in terms of spatial frequency and contrast sensitivity. However, the actual appearance of Seurat's paintings is even more complex because of variations in the visual texture.

In Seurat's works between 1886 and 1891, the distribution of the colored dots on the canvas was very regular. However, the surface of the paintings does not appear entirely uniform, even at a fixed distance of observation. This is not surprising, because, in spite of the regularity of the spatial frequency of the dots, there are important variations in hue, saturation, and lightness from one part of a painting to another. Thus, depending on the part of the painting observed, one's eye can be in the range of contrast, dissociation, assimilation, or optical mixture. Some examples are given in Fig. 11-11. In Fig. 11-11A, the colors are near in hue and lightness and they mix easily, even at a short distance. In Fig. 11-11B, the difference in hues makes optical mixture more difficult. In Fig. 11-11C, there are marked differences in lightness. In Fig. 11-11D, there are differences simultaneously in hue and lightness, making optical mixture very difficult, except at a very great distance. Thus, when the observer varies the distance from the canvas, the appearance of the painting will change in a dramatic fashion, with fluctuations in hue, saturation, and lightness. "This uncertainty, and the lack of distinctness of the different colors," said Brücke, "give the painted surface a certain life which it would not have if covered with an even tint. By this mode of optical mixture, it is possible to obtain visual effects not available in an other way."[10] When the observer moves to clarify the images on the canvas, a contrary event occurs: the painting seems to change with the movement. As Jameson and Hurvich note: "To walk toward and backaway . . . permits one to experience an intriguing change. . . . At a critical range of intermediate viewing distances the variegated grain of the painted surface tends to reach the threshold of resolution without breaking the overall color composition."[11] This variation in optical mixture with visual texture is particularly suited to represent moving appearances of the nature such as shimmering aspects of the foliage; shining reflexes to the surface of running water; and variations of

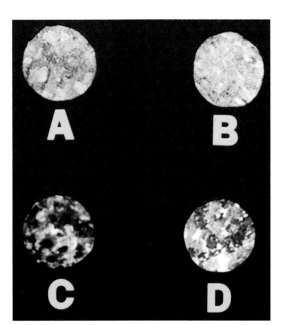

FIGURE **11-11**

Spatial variations of color texture in samples from Seurat's paintings. **A,** Similar hue and lightness. **B,** Hue difference. **C,** Lightness difference. **D,** Both hue and lightness differences. Optical mixture for each of these occurs at a different distance of observation. By changing the viewing distance, it can be demonstrated that samples A and B become fused visually at a shorter distance than samples C and D.

FIGURE 11-12
Seurat. *Port en Bressin, l'Avant Port.*
Oil on canvas, 1888. *(© Photo R.M.N.
Musée d'Orsay, Paris.)*

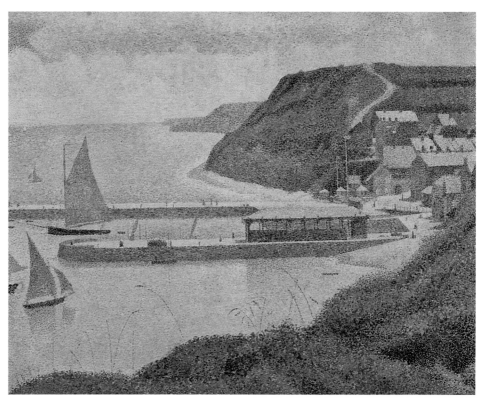

shapes of clouds; of which there are multiple examples in Seurat's works of this period (Fig. 11-12).

CONCLUSIONS

The main innovation of Seurat and pointillism was the marriage of optical mixture and visual texture. Seurat modulated the three attributes of color (hue, saturation, and lightness) by additive optical mixture produced with painted texture. Optical mixture had been used occasionally by some earlier painters in a sporadic fashion, but Seurat made pointillism a systematic discipline and the basic principle of his painting. It should be noted that pointillism differs from the use of larger spots of color, called divisionism by Signac and others. As Ratliff points out, the basis of pointillism was optical mixture, while the basis of divisionism was contrast (and possibly assimilation).[12] Of course, there was no sharp distinction between the two techniques, which were at times practiced by the same artists.

Finally, it is important to emphasize the near impossibility of reproducing Seurat's works, since much of their effect is lost when they are reduced to illustration size. This is unavoidable, for the basis of Seurat's art is the additive mixture of discrete dots in the eye, while the technique of color printing makes colors in a subtractive way. The additive effect explicitly sought by Seurat is replaced by a subtractive mixture, involving all the distortions and darkening of colors inherent to the printing process. For this reason it is with great reluctance that I have included illustrations of paintings in this chapter. At a recent exhibition of the Barnes collection in Paris, I had the opportunity to see *Les Poseuses,* a painting that was previously accessible only in reproduction. Seeing the original was an unforgettable and wonderful revelation. It is possible to obtain faithful reproductions of very small paintings, since one can keep a reasonable point-to-point comparison with the canvas. To appreciate the real effect of Seurat's large works, however, one must go to Chicago for *Un dimanche d'été à la Grande Jatte,* to the Barnes Foundation for *Les poseuses,* and to the Metropolitan Museum in New York for *La Parade*.

REFERENCES

1. Cachin F et al: *Seurat,* Metropolitan Museum of Art, New York, 1991.
2. Gage J: *Colour and culture,* Thames and Hudson, London, 1993.
3 Signac P: *D'Eugène Delacroix au Neo-Impressionisme,* H. Floury, Paris, 1899 (translated by W Silverman as: *From Eugène Delacroix to Neo-Impressionism,* in Ratliff,[12] pp. 193-285; quotations from pp. 248 and 280.)
4. Home WI: *Seurat and the Science of Painting,* MIT Press, Cambridge, Mass., 1964.
5. Minervino F: *Toute l'Oeuvre Peinte de Seurat,* Flammarion, Paris, 1973.
6. Rood O: *Modern Chromatics,* Van Nostrand and Reinhold, New York, 1973 (originally published in 1879).
7. Mullen KT: The chromatic coding of space. In C Blakemore (ed): *Vision: Coding and Efficiency,* Cambridge University Press, Cambridge, Mass., 1990, pp. 150-158.
8. Chevreul ME: *De la Loi du Contraste Simultané des Couleurs.* An English translation by C. Martel: *The Principles of Harmony and Contrast of Colors,* 1854; reprinted by Van Norstrand Reinhold, 1967, New York.
9. Helson H: *Adaption Level Theory,* Harper and Row, New York, 1964.
10. Brücke E: *Des Couleurs au Point de Vue Physique, Physiologique, Artistique et Industriel,* Baillière, 1986.
11. Jameson D, Hurvich LM: From contrast to assimilation: in art and in the eye, *Leonardo* 8:125-131, 1975.
12. Ratliff F: *Paul Signac and Color in Neo-Impressionism.* Rockefeller University Press, New York, 1992.

Part Five

PERSPECTIVE AND ILLUSION

Chapter Twelve

PERSPECTIVE ON PERSPECTIVE

Michael F. Marmor

Perspective seems a natural feature of art to those of us raised in Western culture. We are accustomed to photographic images of the world, in which the depiction of buildings and objects follows strictly the laws of linear perspective relative to the fixed viewing point of the camera lens. Children in school learn how to pick a vanishing point and make buildings look "realistic," and we apply the term "naive" to unschooled painters in whose work perspective is distorted. Indeed, proper perspective almost seems a natural part of the process of seeing, an extension of our vantage point into the world. There is some physiologic truth to this, to the extent that true judgment of depth is only possible because each of our eyes sees the world from a slightly different angle, and our brain is able to analyze these differences as a means of calculating distance. For the most part, however, perspective merely represents the transformation of the three-dimensional world onto a two-dimensional plane held in front of the eye, and while it may represent reality in the sense of a mathematical transfer of images, it does not necessarily or always serve the purpose of art.

Perspective that appears distorted to our Western eyes is not uncommon in art. Distorted or stylized perspective is evident in the art of some ancient cultures, in most of the art of the Middle Ages, in Asian art up to modern times, and in many works of modern artists from Matisse to Hockney. It is tempting to look at paintings from the Renaissance and beyond, which display magnificent perspective, and wonder how it was possible that great painters of earlier eras such as Giotto, or of such countries as China and India, could have failed to recognize the distortion in their works. How could they paint magnificent figures and haunting landscapes but not notice "inconsistencies" that would be picked up by the average modern third grader? We have no evidence that the eye has changed over the past few millennia, and in fact the use of perspective was quite sophisticated in ancient Greece and Rome (Fig. 12-1). Trompe l'oeil (fool the eye) wall paintings were used in many of the villas of Pompeii to enhance the architecture and give an illusion of space. In other words, careful observers throughout history have been able to produce reasonable (if not necessarily mathematical) perspective, although this technique was utilized rather selectively.

Did artists who ignored perspective do so for lack of interest or skill, for failure to perceive their "errors," or for a desire or need to portray different elements of information in their work? I would suggest that the last of these is most likely, and this notion is supported by evidence that artistic conventions have existed throughout the history of art. Even in the ancient world, philosophers argued about whether art should be representational and whether perspective was valid. In a famous passage, Plato wrote: "You may look at a bed or any other object from straight in front or slantwise or at any angle. Is there any difference in the bed itself, or does it merely look different? . . . Does painting aim at reproducing any actual object as it is, or the appearance of it as it looks? In other words, is it a representation of the truth or of a semblance? . . . The are of representation, then, is a long way from reality.[1] In fairness, Plato is judging art against his philosophical ideal of truth and reality rather than as an aesthetic endeavor, but the passage shows clearly that people in ancient times were no less aware of these issues than we are today.

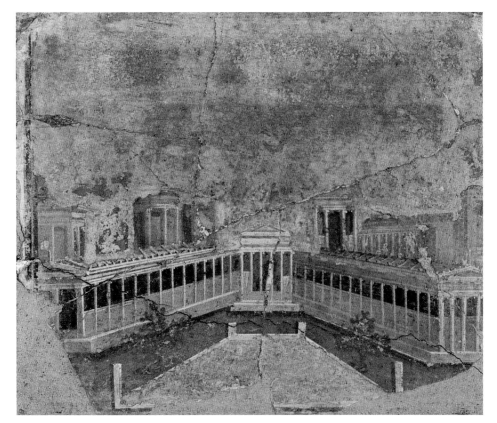

FIGURE 12-1

Anonymous. *View of a Villa.*

Roman architectural wall painting from Pompeii, c. 60 B.C., showing elements of linear perspective. (*Museo Archeologico Nazionale, Naples, Italy.* [*Scala/Art Resource, NY.*])

Artists in earlier eras were generally required (by those who hired them) to convey not only images but also a message. In this context, perspective becomes only one technique among many for "selling the product," which might by a religious belief, a ruler's spin on history, or a record of wealthy man's property for his tomb. In ancient Egypt, figures were painted in a flat and stylized manner (Fig. 12-2), with the head forward, the eye looking sideways, the chest facing the viewer (although nipple and umbilicus may face forward), the feet heading forward, and so on. It is doubtful that any of us not working as a contortionist could duplicate this stance, but to the Egyptians it clearly provided essential facts about each subject. The Egyptians were no strangers to three-dimensional representation, as evidenced by their magnificent sculptures, but they seemed unconcerned about lack of realism in their paintings and reliefs. It was only important that pictures tell the story for which they were commissioned. One may surmise that a similar rationale lies behind the curious loss of perspective when the Greek and Roman civilizations faded and Western Europe entered the Dark Ages: Byzantine painting (Fig. 12-3) focused on religious figures and stories, for which the message was paramount and the scenic background was secondary. Sometimes the same character even appeared several times in one picture to illustrate a narrative sequence. The purpose of these pictures was not to serve as a "postcard" illustrating heaven for those who had not yet made the trip but rather to serve as a vehicle for teaching gospel beliefs that were in fact beyond the real world. The message became the medium, and it would have been undesirable to distract the viewer with irrelevant realism.

It has always seemed curious to me that perspective, which seems such a natural process for reproducing on canvas what we see in the world, was either lost or consciously omitted from art for centuries—and then reappeared with a

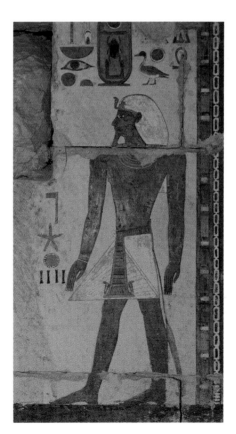

FIGURE **12-2**
Thutmose III. Temple of Hatshepsut,
Luxor-Thebes, Egypt.
(Borromeo/Art Resource, NY.)

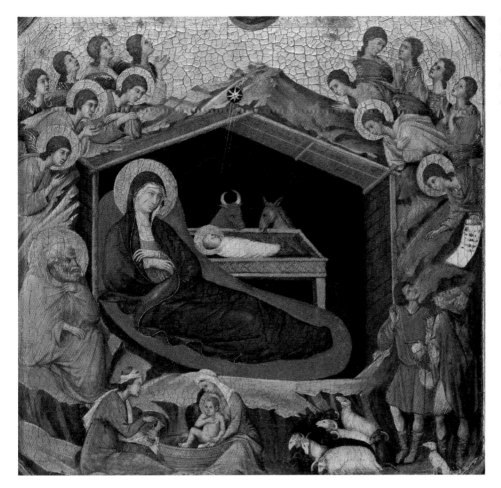

vengeance within the space of just a few years in the early part of the fifteenth century.[2,3] The Italian masters of the late 1300s had begun to explore the limited use of perspective, but they still focused primarily on subject rather than architectural precision. Around 1420, the great Florentine architect Brunelleschi (who later built the dome of the grand cathedral in Florence) devised a "demonstration" in which he made an accurate illusionistic painting of the baptistery, as viewed from the door of the cathedral. A viewer who stood at the proper spot and looked through a peephole could hardly tell if the scene was real or the perspective painting. The impact of this technique was enormous, perhaps because the cultural and political changes of the Renaissance made the public (and the church) more worldly and scientific so that realism could be accepted (and even demanded) in art. Within a decade Masaccio had painted his famous *Trinity* on the wall of Santa Maria Novella church, which gave the illusion of a chapel receding into the wall (Fig. 12-4), and by 1435 another architect-painter, Leon Battista Alberti, wrote his famous treatise *On Painting*, which provided a do-it-yourself manual for creating a vanishing point and the receding rays of linear perspective. Word traveled fast, and by the mid-1400s all of the major Italian painters were using linear perspective. Indeed, some paintings (Fig. 12-5) were virtual treatises in perspective technique, in addition to (or sometimes to the exclusion of) other artistic merits. The love for perspective almost got out of hand in the ensuing centuries, when painters like Canaletto and Saenredam constructed large and complex views of cities, cathedrals, and other structural entities to highlight the power of perspective in generating an illusion of space. Those illusions could be

FIGURE   12-4
Masaccio. *The Trinity.*
c. 1427. Santa Maria Novella, Florence,
Italy. Compare with the Roman wall
painting created 1500 years earlier.
(Erich Lessing/Art Resource, NY.)

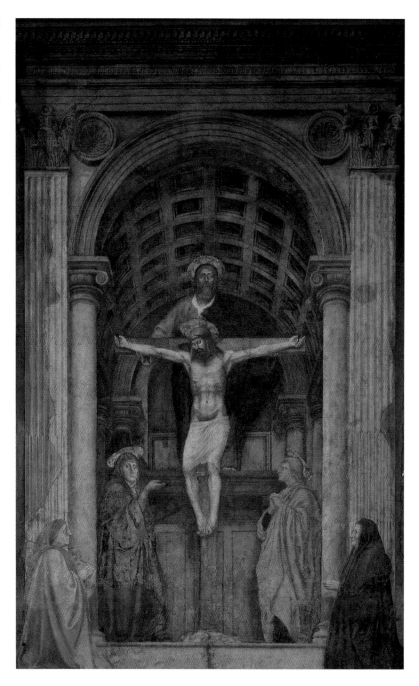

so powerful that Baroque architects placed perspective murals on the low-domed
ceilings of many churches (Fig. 12-6) to give a sense of space and height (and to
avoid the cost of building a higher dome).

Although a perspective view may seem representative of true vision, it is at the
same time artificial. A perspective painting represents a scene from only a single
fixed point of view, like one frame out of a motion picture. Many artists such as
Picasso (Fig. 12-7) and Hockney (Fig. 12-8) have tried to illustrate the fact that
natural vision is always moving and scanning by creating distorted or multiple
images. Picasso's striking *Portrait of Dora Maar* shows both front and side views,
simulating the reality that no person exists only in profile. Hockney has put these
concerns into words as well as art: "Perspective makes you think of deep space on

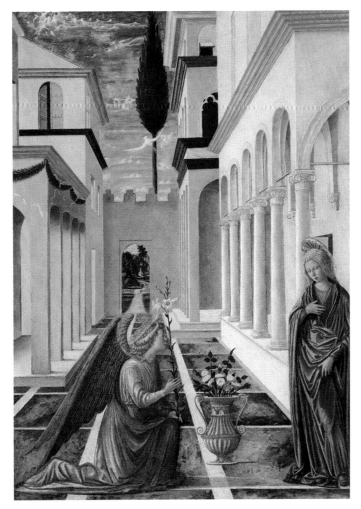

FIGURE   12-5
Master of the Panels.
The Annunciation.
c. 1450. *(Samuel H. Kress Collection,
©1996 Board of Trustees, National
Gallery of Art, Washington D.C.)*

a flat surface. But the trouble with perspective is that it has no movement at all. The one vanishing point exists for only a fraction of a second to us. . . My point about the desk photograph is that if you are seeing around the corners of the desk, you are seeing yourself move. It isn't just the desk, it is you and the desk. You are united with it, in the process of looking. You are aware of yourself in space."[2]

Even the finest perspective image will appear distorted when viewed from an "incorrect" vantage point. This effect is accentuated with architectural trompe l'oeil paintings, which is the reason Brunelleschi required his viewers to use a specific peephole. The trompe l'oeil ceiling paintings in churches give a wonderful sense of height when you can stand at the exact center of the floor, but from the side of the church one sees strangely tilted structures and figures (see Fig. 12-6). Hoogstraten painted scenes on the interior walls of boxes that look bizarre viewed from the front but show a precisely drawn scene through a peephole on one wall. This distortion of objects to compensate for oblique views is called anamorphism. Holbein's great painting of the ambassadors (in the National Gallery in London) has a curious elongated object near the bottom that is seen to be a skull when viewed at a very shallow angle through a peephole in the frame of the painting. The same technique allows one to decipher William Scrots' portrait of Edward VI shown in Fig. 12-9. The use of anamorphic projections is not totally a game, however, since there are places in ordinary life where we cannot avoid an angled view: look, for example, at the elongated letters in "STOP" or "YIELD" signs painted on the street.

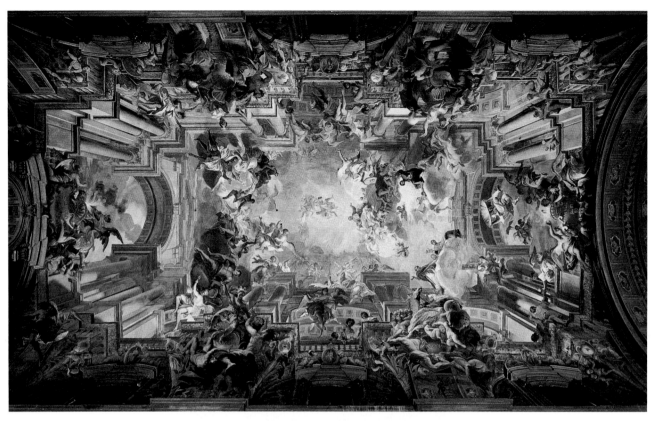

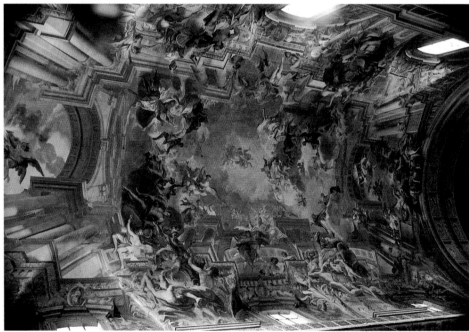

FIGURE **12-6**

Pozzo. *Ascension of*
St. Ignatius into Paradise.
Ceiling fresco. 1691-1694. S. Ignazio,
Rome, Italy. **Top:** Viewed properly,
from a disk on the floor, from which
the full view was photographed, the
ceiling appears high above, supported
by full columns. However, these
features are all painted. **Bottom**:
If the ceiling is viewed from the
wrong part of the church, as in the
detail, distortion becomes obvious.
(Scala/Art Resource, NY.)

Despite the visual impact of perspective as used in Western art, quite different conventions of perspective are found in the art of China and Japan and in traditional Islamic art. Asian brush paintings (Fig. 12-10) are characteristically flat in appearance, with distances indicated by overlap between objects, by height on the paper, or by progressive haze (atmospheric perspective). Both size cues and convergent perspective are used only to a limited degree. As in ancient Egypt, this

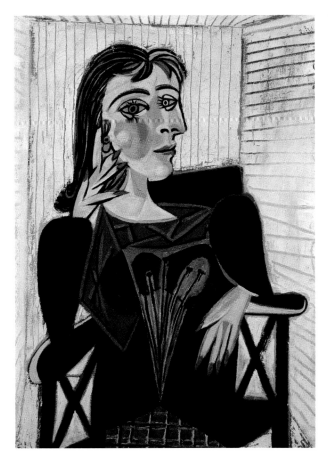

FIGURE 12-7
Picasso. *Portrait of Dora Maar.*
Oil, 1937. (Copyright 1996 Estate of Pablo Picasso/Artists Rights Society [ARS] New York. Musée Picasso, Paris, France. [Giraudon/Art Resource, NY.])

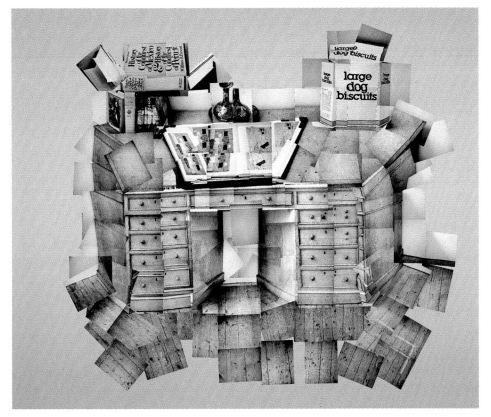

FIGURE 12-8
Hockney. *The Desk.*
July 1st, 1984. Photographic collage, © David Hockney.

FIGURE 12-9
Scrots. *Edward VI.*
1546. **Top:** Anamorphic view.
Bottom: The proper view, taken
photographically at a very oblique
angle through the indentation frame.
This can be mimicked by tilting the
page to look at the anamorphism
from a very oblique angle.
*(Courtesy of The National Portrait
Gallery, London.)*

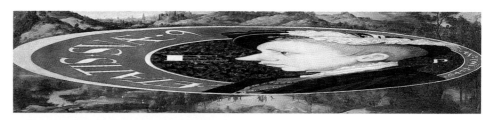

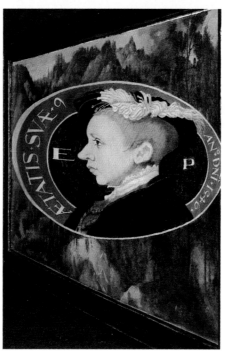

style was understood by its culture, and it conveyed the information desired without regard for whether it represented reality. The artists told a story, imparted a sense of emotion, or illustrated a characteristic of nature rather than nature itself.

In some of these brush paintings, but more striking in work from the Islamic and Indian empires, one sees objects drawn in "reverse perspective," in other words, drawn so that parallel lines *diverge* with distance (Fig. 12-11). Divergent perspective is also seen in many Western paintings from the Middle Ages (see Fig. 12-3), in ancient primitive art, and in modern "naive" paintings. How does one explain this technique, which seems not merely a deviation from, but a total controversion of, visual experience? First, or course, we come back to earlier arguments that art is not necessarily representational and that we must inquire as to what information the artist is trying to convey. As Plato argued, a bed will be the same no matter how it is viewed, and thus a rectangular or divergent image may serve an artist's purpose better than a perspective image if it provides more room on which to draw the design of the bedspread or show the occupants of the bed. Linear perspective gives a sense of three-dimensionality, but it also reduces the amount of detail one can show of distant objects because of their shrinking size. One motivation for neutral or divergent perspective may be a desire to give equal importance, or equal detail, to objects at different depths within the scene.

Deregowski and Parker[5] have pointed out that divergent perspective may also reflect some aspects of normal perception, depending on the angle with which objects are viewed. As shown in Fig. 12-12, objects that are off to one side occupy a larger visual angle far away than when they are up close, even though in a

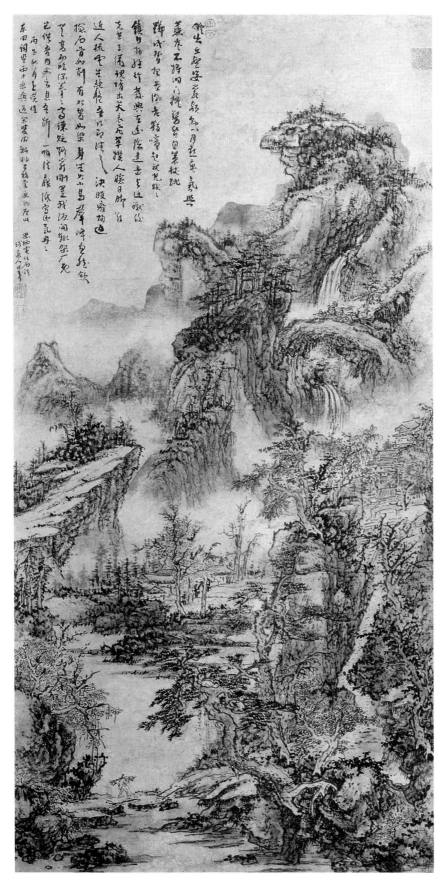

FIGURE   12-11
Bicitr (attributed). *Shah Shuja Enthroned with Gaj Singh of Marwar.* Mughal, c. 1638. Reverse perspective in Indian art. *(Los Angeles County Museum of Art, The Nasli and Alice Heeramaneck collection, Museum Associates Purchase.)*

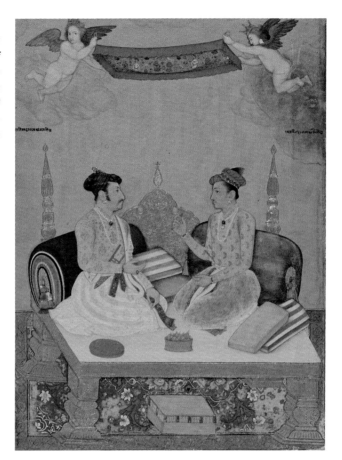

FIGURE   12-12
Diagram of perspective convergence and divergence, depending on the position of an object. When an object (*O*) recedes in front of an observer, the visual angle it subtends will diminish as it gets farther away (angle *a* is less than angle *b*). However, if the object is far off to one side, the visual angle will *increase* as the object recedes (angle *c* is greater than angle *d*). Faraway objects will always be smaller in the plane of a picture (i.e., as drawn with linear perspective) but not necessarily on the retina. *(Modified from Deregowski JB, Parker DM.[5])*

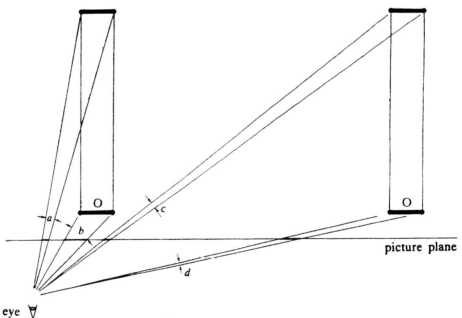

picture plane (i.e., using linear perspective) the faraway object will be smaller. A larger visual angle means that a larger portion of retina is stimulated, so there is a true expansion of size. Awareness of this phenomenon may have contributed at times to an artist's choice of divergent perspective, although it seems doubtful that this peculiarity of side vision explains the consistent use of divergent per-

There are interesting data from animal experiments that bear on this issue. When kittens are raised inside an enclosure that contains only vertical stripes (and no horizontal elements), the cells in their brain lose the ability to recognize horizontals.[8] Thus, it is not inconceivable that children raised in environments that are singularly lacking in certain visual elements could be less capable physically of recognizing them. On the other hand, it is hard to assess whether the real world can ever provide a sufficiently skewed visual input for this effect to be significant. It has been argued that the "carpentered" world of Western society helps youngsters to recognize right angles and perspective representations relative to individuals raised in a forest or plain where there are no boxlike structures. However, even nature is dominated by verticals (trees and cliffs) and horizontals (the ground and horizon), so it would be surprising to find major organic differences in visual capability even among groups living in disparate environments. Culture and environment may under certain circumstances influence the perception of perspective, but even if present such an effect would be only one factor among many that interact to determine how individuals create art, perceive art, and use art.[9,10,11]

While linear perspective in painting is an important artistic tool that mimics a photographic view of the world, it is not the only tool for evoking a sense of depth. Awareness of depth is achieved through many visual (and artistic) cues such as size of familiar objects, the covering of one object by another, the fading of colors with distance, and shadows. People who have lost one eye have surprisingly little difficulty functioning in our society, despite their lack of true depth perception, because they use these other cues quite automatically. Some of these cues, such as overlap of objects and atmospheric haze over distant objects, are often used in lieu of linear perspective, especially in Asian art (see Fig. 12-9). The presence of shadows, however, is so linked to realism in artistic representation that their appearance has to a large degree matched the use of perspective. For example, shadows are found in many Roman wall paintings but are absent from Egyptian painting and from the iconographic art in the Middle Ages. They began to appear again in paintings from the early Renaissance, but they were represented accurately only as linear perspective was perfected. This omission of shadows in most nonperspective art supports the thesis that perspective has been used (or avoided) more for reasons of convention or style than for lack of observation or skill, since no special geometric techniques are needed to place a shadow behind a person standing in the sun.

Some modern artists are drifting away again from the use of linear perspective, as they seek out new purposes and new ways for art to stimulate the viewer without arbitrary constraints of technique. Where art functions for the purpose of illustration, perspective is essential; however, where art tells a story, conveys emotion, or shocks the senses, perspective may divert attention to secondary features of the painting. In Hockney's photomontages (see Fig. 12-8), the multiple exposures simulate the reality that our eyes cannot hold absolutely still or see anything from a single vantage point. Were such pictures painted conventionally in perfect perspective, we might be drawn to admire the construction of the objects instead of their visual and psychological significance. Picasso's tender rendering of *Paolo Drawing* (Fig. 12-16) includes a desk of rather peculiar shape and tilt, but the open surface allows one to see Paolo's youthful scribbles, which are more important than the architecture of the furniture. Anyone who has attended a movie in recent years is aware that form and space are now moldable through computer manipulation, and our societal attraction to rectilinear representations may become less rigid in the years to come. The facts of photographic perspective are immutable; but the role of perspective in art may be best understood as a matter of perspective.

FIGURE 12-16

Picasso. *Paolo Drawing.*

Oil, 1923. *(©1996 Estate of Pablo Picasso/Artists Rights Society [ARS], New York. Musée Picasso, Paris, France. Giraudon/Art Resource, NY.)*

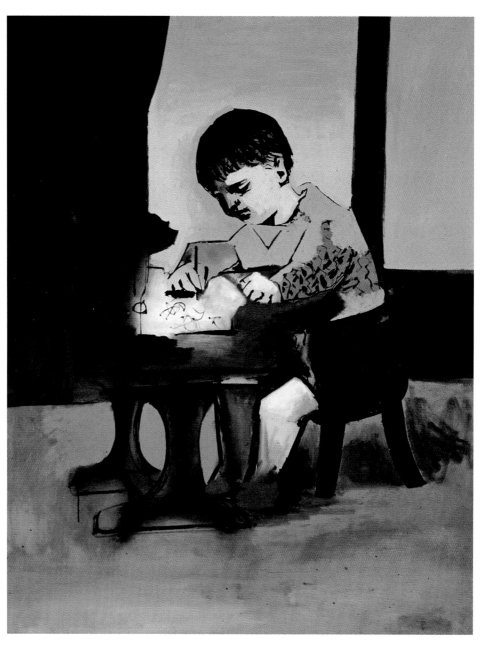

FIGURE 12-16

Picasso. *Paolo Drawing.*

Oil, 1923. *(©1996 Estate of Pablo Picasso/Artists Rights Society [ARS], New York. Musée Picasso, Paris, France. Giraudon/Art Resource, NY.)*

— **REFERENCES** —

1. Plato: *The Republic*, Oxford University Press, New York, 1945, p. 328 (Book X) (translated by FM Cornford).
2. Wright L: *Perspective in Perspective*. Routledge & Kegan Paul, London, 1983.
3. White J: *The Birth and Rebirth of Pictorial Space*. Balknap (Harvard), Cambridge, 1987.
4. Hockney D: *Hockney on Photography. Conversations with Paul Joyce*. Jonathan Cope, London, 1988, pp. 30, 140.
5. Deregowski JB, Parker DM: Convergent and divergent perspective, *Perception* 21:441-447, 1992.
6. Hudson W: Pictorial depth perception in sub-cultural groups in Africa, *J Soc Psychol* 52:183-208, 1960.
7. Deregowski JB: Real space and represented space: Cross-cultural perspectives, *Behav Brain Sci* 12:51-119, 1989.
8. Blakemore C: Development of the brain depends on the visual environment, *Nature* 228:477-488, 1970.
9. Gombrich EH: *Art and Illusion*. Princeton University Press, Princeton, 1960.
10. Arnheim R: *Art and Visual Perception*. University of California Press, Berkeley, 1974.
11. Deregowski JB: *Illusions, Patterns and Pictures*. Academic Press, London, 1980.

Chapter Thirteen

ILLUSION AND OPTICAL ART

Michael F. Marmor

Pictorial representation is by nature somewhat illusory. Perspective is designed to fool us into seeing a three-dimensional world on a two-dimensional canvas, and philosophers as far back as Plato (see Chapter 12) have argued over the wisdom of such artifice. However, representation is not the only purpose of art, and through the ages paintings have served to document, inform, educate, indoctrinate, record, emote, and occasionally shock. Most notable in modern times, paintings have been created solely for their visual effect independent of other contexts. Some of these works have been called optical art (or op art). In this breadth of roles for art, illusion is no longer just a device to create a sense of depth or space; in some cases it becomes the image itself. Psychologists and art historians have debated for centuries about the role or importance of illusion in art, and visual scientists have struggled to explain and classify visual illusions.[1] Books that have been written on the subject include the wonderful monographs by Arnheim[2] and Gombrich.[3] These issues will not be resolved in the space of a few pages, and my purpose is simply to offer a framework for thinking about visual illusions (and why they work in the eye and in art). I hope this framework will provide some insight or encouragement to appreciate this visual aspect of art.

Visual illusions are, by definition, phenomena that fool us. However, one could argue about whether the definition should be fool the eye or fool the brain. The distinction is quite important, if one interprets the word "brain" to include the psychologic components of how we recognize, interpret, and appreciate things. The eye, of course, can only respond to images in a physical way with circuits that are hardwired essentially the same way in all people. This is the hardware in our visual computer. Conscious visual perception, however, is influenced by what we have learned by peer pressure, by interest, and by attention. The enormous power of the brain to recognize, interpret, and appreciate objects represents software in our visual computer—and some individuals process with WordPerfect while others choose Write Now.

To the extent that we can recognize hardware and software components of visual perception, we can also recognize illusions that depend on hardwired circuitry and illusions that depend primarily on softwired acculturation or experience. Some illusions bridge the gap and depend on a mixture of hardwired and softwired mechanisms, but the dichotomy can still be helpful in understanding their impact in art.

HARDWIRED ILLUSIONS

Perhaps the most prevalent example of a hardwired illusory phenomenon is the Mach band, which represents an enhancement of perceived contrast at edges (see Chapter 6). Mach bands are a perceptual manifestation of the fact that the retina and primary visual pathways are designed to emphasize contrast between light and dark as a means of simplifying and coding visual images. The number of nerve fibers between eye and brain is much smaller than the number of photoreceptor elements in the retina, and as visual information converges on these nerve fibers the circuitry automatically enhances the response to contrast while minimizing the response to diffuse light or darkness. Thus, the perception of illusions based on Mach bands or similar contrast phenomena is inherent in the human species. Mach bands appear in many types of art, as discussed in Chapter 6, and although you can learn from experience to recognize them and to make judgments carefully where they might cause confusion, the illusion is always there for the young and old, for the naive and sophisticated.

A related illusion is the Hermann grid, shown in Fig. 13-1. When looking at this pattern of white lines on a dark background, you see evanescent gray spots at the intersections of the white lines; they disappear curiously whenever you look directly at them. These fleeting spots are thought to arise from the center-surround organization of the retinal bipolar and ganglion cells (see Chapter 1). The figure shows diagrammatically that the center of each intersection will appear darker because there is more inhibitory input to the cells whose receptive field is centered on the intersection. But why do the dark spots disappear when you look right at them? The answer lies in the fact that the center of our retina is specialized for sharp vision while our side vision is rather fuzzy and serves mainly for orientation and the detection of motion. The receptive fields for each cell in the center of our retina are very tiny (to enable us to read fine print) but get larger away from center. As you look directly at an intersection, the tiny receptive fields of your central vision fall entirely within the white space, so there is no difference between line and intersection. Only in off-center vision, where the center-surround areas are large enough to correspond to the width of the lines, does the Hermann grid phenomenon appear. These evanescent spots are hard to find in classical painting amidst complex shapes and images. However modern artists such as Vasarely have constructed images whose fascination and vibrancy are in part a result of these inescapable fleeting spots (Fig. 13-2).

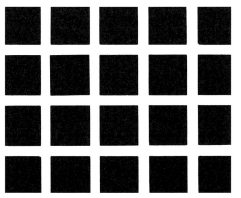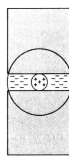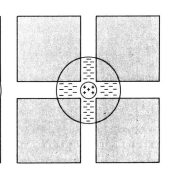

FIGURE 13-1
Hermann grid. Evanescent gray spots are perceived at the intersections of the white lines. The diagram shows a proposed explanation for the phenomenon. At each intersection there is twice as much light on the inhibitory surround region of the receptive fields of the retinal neurons.

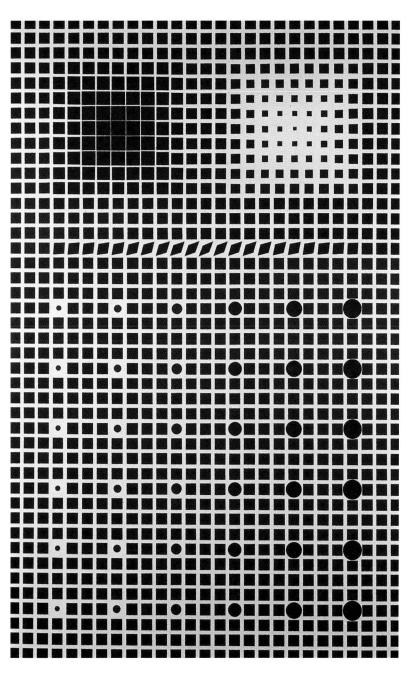

FIGURE 13-2
Vasarely. *Supernovae.*
Oil, 1959-1961. *(Copyright 1996 Artist Rights Society [ARS], New York/ADAGP, Paris. Tate Gallery, London/Art Resource, NY.)*

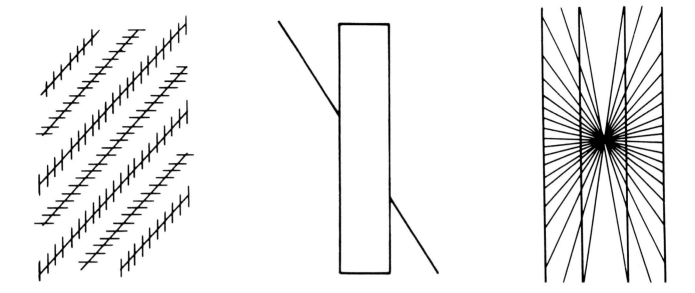

FIGURE 13-3

Three illusions of direction. **Left:** Zöllner illusion. The longer lines do not appear parallel. **Middle:** Poggendorff illusion. The broken line does not appear continuous. **Right:** Hering illusion. The central lines do not appear parallel.

Some illusions (Fig. 13-3) depend on distortion of our sense of directionality when angled lines impinge upon a straight line. In the Zöllner illusion, for example, parallel lines appear to diverge or converge, depending on the direction of the angled cross-hatching. A single line drawn at an angle to a rectangular bar (Poggendorff illusion) seems to show displacement of the two segments. In the Hering illusion, parallel lines that cross a set of radiations appear to bulge. The origin of these illusions is unknown but may involve a component of experience or acculturation insofar as they evoke some memory of familiar objects or shapes. However, it is also quite likely that these phenomena depend on the interaction of visual cortical cells that are specialized for directional sensitivity (see Chapter 1). The brain has the ability to combine information from hundreds or thousands of directionally sensitive cells to see "straightness" of a line, or to interpret the significance of an angled junction. When the continuum is interrupted by a gap (as in the Poggendorff illusion), or is so overloaded with information (as with the angled lines in the Zöllner and Hering illusions), the interpretations may become biased as the brain attempts to integrate all of this information into a cohesive scheme. These illusions contribute to the complex effects of Bridget Riley's *Descending* (Fig. 13-4).

Another part of the effect of *Descending* comes from the juxtaposition of very closely spaced lines. It is difficult to hold fixation while looking at this pattern, so it seems to move or shimmer. The physiologic basis of this effect is the requirement that our eyes be moving a little bit all the time, because absolutely stable images on the retina would fade out within seconds. Retinal cells require contrast to stimulate them, and to provide this our eyes are continuously in motion with a very fine quivering that we do not consciously recognize. This property of vision has been exploited not only by modern op artists like Anuszkiewicz (Fig. 13-5) but also by others intrigued with the visual effects. Navaho weavers make "eye-dazzler" rugs that juxtapose colors in patterns so fine that image shimmers (Fig. 13-6), and the patterns on some Indian pottery are equally evocative. The Acoma seed pot design shown in Fig. 13-7 shimmers and the lines arcing out from the core create ambiguity between circles and spirals in the intersecting pattern. Zeki and Lamb found that one of the secondary visual cortical areas in the brain (area V5) contains cells that respond selectively to movement and direction, and thus it is specialized for the perception of motion. When they measured brain activity

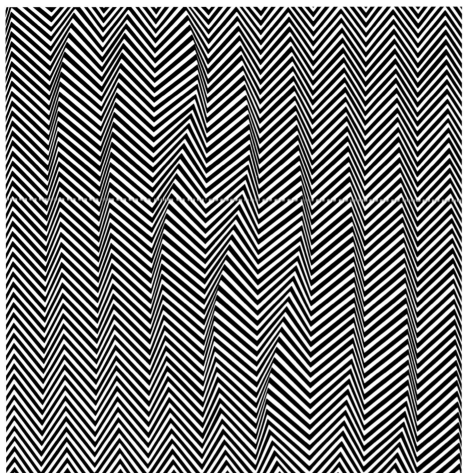

FIGURE 13-4

Riley. *Descending.*
Emulsion on board, 1965-1966.
(Private collection, London.)

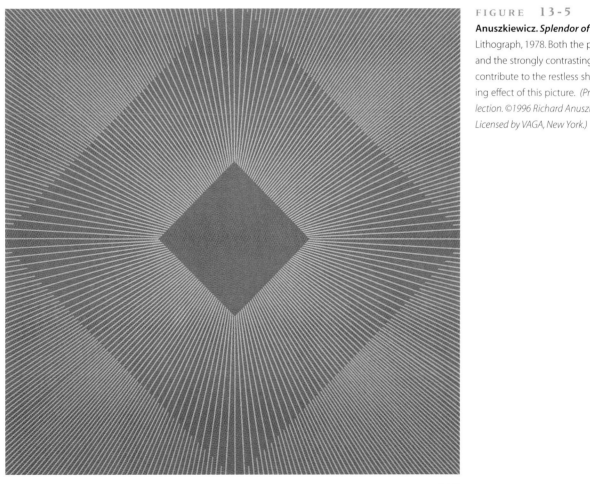

FIGURE 13-5

Anuszkiewicz. *Splendor of Orange.*
Lithograph, 1978. Both the pattern
and the strongly contrasting colors
contribute to the restless shimmering effect of this picture. *(Private collection. ©1996 Richard Anuszkiewicz/
Licensed by VAGA, New York.)*

FIGURE **13-6**

M. Benally. Woven Navajo rug, 1992. *(Tec Nos Pos, Arizona. Private collection.)*

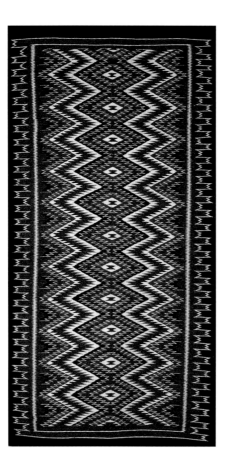

FIGURE **13-7**

B. Cerno and J. Cerno. Seed pot, 1989. *(Acoma Pueblo, New Mexico. Private collection.)*

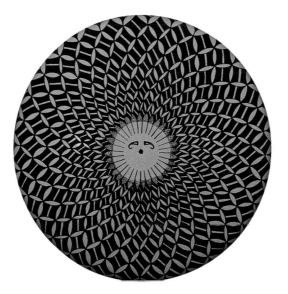

while subjects looked at pictures that showed illusory movement, they found that the activity localized in the V5 region. Thus, specific brain regions can be critical for perceiving illusory effects in art (and in life). They caution, however, that these observations "do not . . . imply that the resulting aesthetic experience is due solely to the activity of V5 but only that V5 is necessary for it."[4]

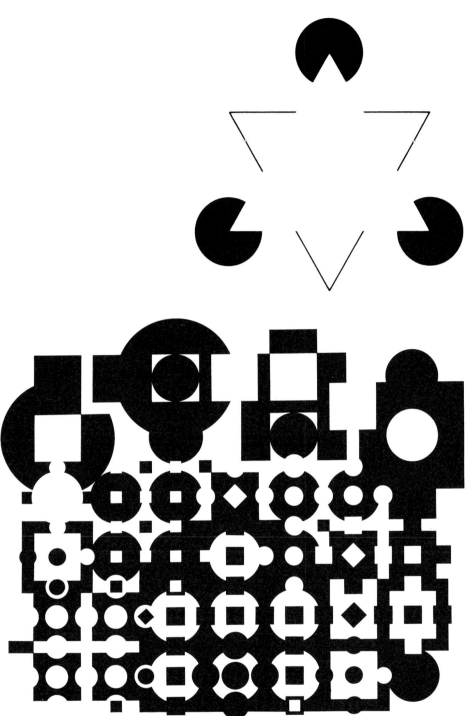

FIGURE   13-8

Kanizsa triangle. A white triangle is seen, although no lines define it.

FIGURE   13-9

Vasarely. *Hélios*.

Oil, 1960. Partial forms create illusory shapes much like the Kanizsa triangle. *(©1996 Artists Rights Society [ARS], New York/ADAGP, Paris.)*

Another set of illusions that may invoke hardwired circuitry are those that produce illusory contours. A classic example is the Kanizsa triangle (Fig. 13-8): one perceives a well-defined white triangle between the three corner wedges, although there are no border lines and the figure is essentially a figment of the imagination. A number of modern artists, including Albers, Riley, and Vasarely (Fig. 13-9), have made paintings that invoke this illusion, causing one to perceive lines where none actually exists. The origin of these illusions is not fully understood. Undoubtedly some of these perceptions derive from our experiential famil-

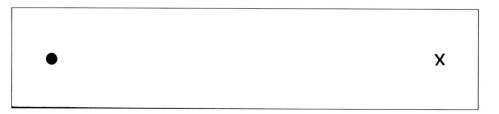

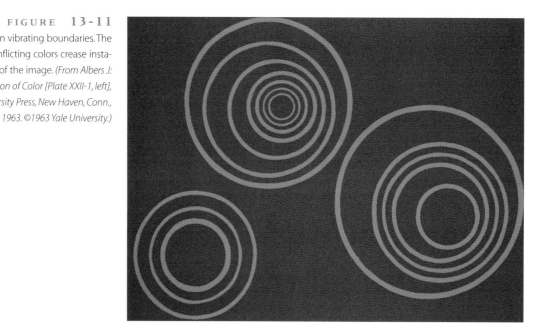

iarity with shapes and our tacit assumption that every drawing is trying to show a real object. However, part of the illusion may derive from a fundamental characteristic of our visual system: the tendency to fill in space from border information. The fact that information from every photoreceptor cannot be transmitted unmodified to the brain requires visual information to be simplified, and one mechanism by which the eye and brain accomplish this is to minimize the expenditure of neural energy on images that do not change.

An example of this phenomenon is the blind spot in everyone's eye that corresponds to the place where the optic nerve fibers enter the eye (Fig. 13-10). The most interesting thing about the blind spot is the fact that we never notice it. Even if you look about with one eye closed, you cannot perceive a gap in ordinary images unless you carefully watch for a specific object to disappear. Charles II of England, the "merry monarch," is reported to have amused himself by looking about this way to see what his courtiers would look like without their heads (a somewhat ironic game, of course, since his father, Charles I, had been beheaded by Cromwell).[5] The eminent neuroscientist, K.S. Lashley, performed similar nefarious experiments to "decapitate" irritating dinner companions.[6] He also suffered from occasional migraines in which his central vision would temporarily black out and produce a large blind spot. During one of these attacks he looked at a friend and was shocked to find that not only had the head disappeared but the wallpaper pattern had filled in the blank space and extended down to the collar.[7] It was as if Lashley had suddenly obtained x-ray vision. However, there is another explanation for this phenomenon. In the absence of any new edges or

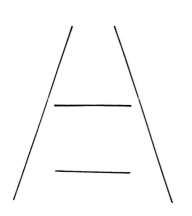 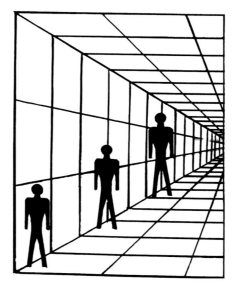

FIGURE 13-12

Illusions of perspective and size. **Left**, Ponzo illusion. The upper bar appears larger. **Right**, Perspective drawing giving the illusion that the figures increase progressively in size.

contrasts to interrupt the wallpaper pattern, the brain automatically extended "perception" of the pattern through the blind spot until the first new or different image was recognized.[8]

Some of the color effects in op art may also derive from hardwired physiologic properties of vision. Fig. 13-11 shows a work by Albers in which bluish green circles lie on a bright orange-red background. Color information is processed in the retina and brain by cells that are specialized for the recognition of color contrasts, particularly between red and green and between blue and yellow (see Chapter 1). These color juxtapositions have special significance, therefore, insofar as they represent intrinsically conflicting sensations. This same painting in green and yellow, or purple and blue, would be interesting but would lack the vibrancy and disturbing contrast that reflects the separation of red and green within the nervous system. Color contrast also contributes to the vibrancy and the shimmer of the Anuszkiewicz lithograph in Fig. 13-5.

SOFTWIRED ILLUSIONS

In contrast to the illusions described above, there are illusory phenomena that seem dependent primarily on past experience or expectations. The prototypes are illusions based on perspective, such as the Ponzo illusion or the illusion of the man in the tunnel (Fig. 13-12). Here our perception that the second bar or second figure is larger than the first is a direct result of our assumption that the angled lines signify receding space. As noted elsewhere (see Chapter 12) such perspective illusions are sometimes less effective for individuals raised in a primitive culture who have not seen photographs or perspective drawings. One could argue that much of art is dominated by perspective illusions, either as a device used to enhance the sense of the reality or as a device omitted (such as in Byzantine, Egyptian, or Asian art) to focus our attention on other meanings such as religious symbolism, documentation of events, or the transmittal of an emotional sensation. Modern op artists have exploited our strong Western sense of perspective, and our strong expectations of "seeing" objects in art, to make paintings that explicitly play on our sensations and our expectations. The sensuous bulge of the Vasarely shown in Fig. 13-13 occurs because our experience and our sense of perspective makes us see three-dimensionality in the image rather than just a pattern of colors and shapes. Perspective illusions are not limited to op art. The forest scene in Munch's *Yellow Log* (Fig. 13-14) is a favorite of school children who visit the Munch Museum in Oslo. It shows cut logs in the snow, and as you move from one side of the picture to the other, the central log seems to move so that its end is always pointing toward you. This illusion depends on our interpretation of, and expectations from, the pictorial clues that make the log appear like a real object in space. If we were to walk to the right or left in the actual forest, we would recognize changes in the scene (e.g., an interjection of trees, and more or less visibility of the sides of the log) that tell us the log has a fixed position in space. However, when we move in front of this painting none of these real world changes take place. The same standing trees still frame a space about the log, and the log still seems to recede in the general direction of our gaze. Because our gaze shifts in direction as we move sideways in front of the picture, so must the apparent position of the log. The same effect probably accounts for the eerie sensation that many painted portraits seem to follow us with their eyes. The amount of white of the eye that is visible on either side of the pupil would change if we walked past an individual whose gaze remained fixed straight ahead. The amount of white remains fixed in a painting, however, so that the eyes seem always to point toward us—and thus appear to follow us as we walk by.

Other softwired illusions that depend on experience and expectation are those of impossible figures and ambiguity. The classic ambiguous figure is the Necker cube (Fig. 13-15) that may be visualized in two orientations. It has formed the basis of art for millennia and was a frequent design in Greco-Roman mosaics (Fig. 13-16). The Albers drawing in Fig. 13-17 is fascinating because the image appears

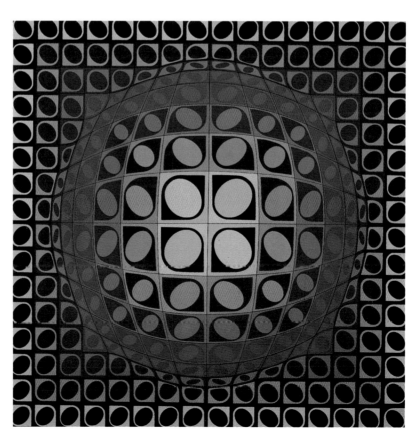

both impossible (it is not easily constructed in reality) and ambiguous (it seems to oscillate in and out of different planes). The impossible triangle and never-ending staircase of Penrose and Penrose (Fig. 13-18)[9] have been immortalized artistically by Escher who transformed the triangle into a magical scene of perpetually falling water (Fig. 13-19). The Vasarely image in Fig. 6-10 is also an impossible object, as is the familiar trident in Fig. 12-15. All of these illusions depend on our innate desire to find real and familiar objects in what we see.

Illusions in which the role of acculturation is probable, but less certain, are those that involve misjudgment of length or size (Fig. 13-20). In the Müller-Lyon

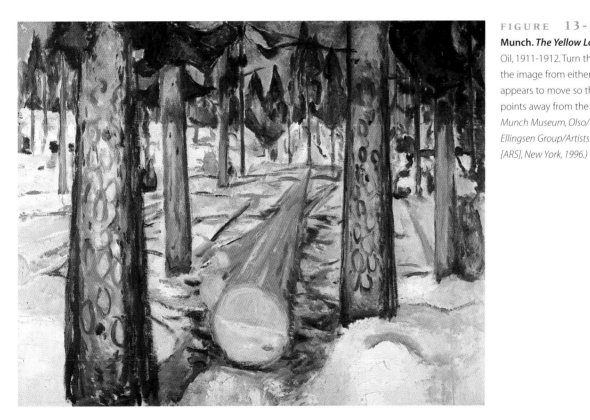

FIGURE 13-14

Munch. *The Yellow Log.*

Oil, 1911-1912. Turn the page to view the image from either side; the log appears to move so that it always points away from the mover. (© *The Munch Museum, Olso/The Munch-Ellingsen Group/Artists Rights Society [ARS], New York, 1996.*)

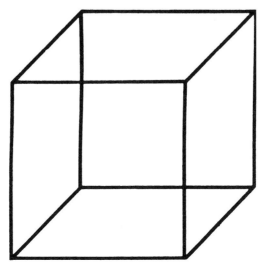

FIGURE 13-15

Necker cube, an ambiguous object. A structure can be seen in two different orientations.

FIGURE   **13-16**
Mosaic design. House of Trajan's
Aqueduct at Antioch. 2nd century
A.D. *(Photograph from the Department
of Art and Archeology, Princeton
University.)*

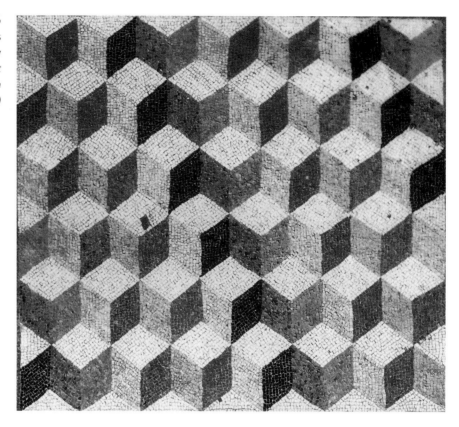

FIGURE   **13-17**
Albers. *Structural Constellations.*
1953-1958. This design is both
ambiguous and impossible as a
physical object. *(Reproduced courtesy
of the Josef and Anni Albers
Foundation.)*

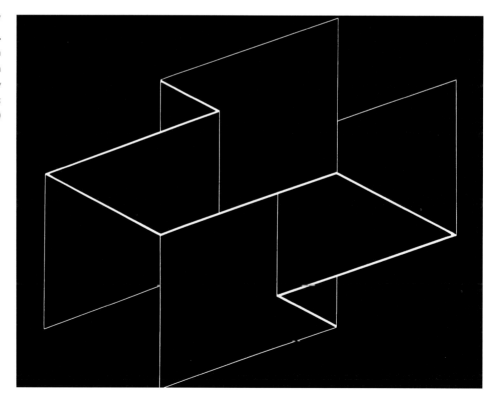

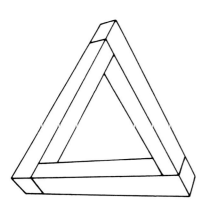 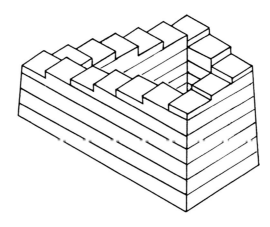

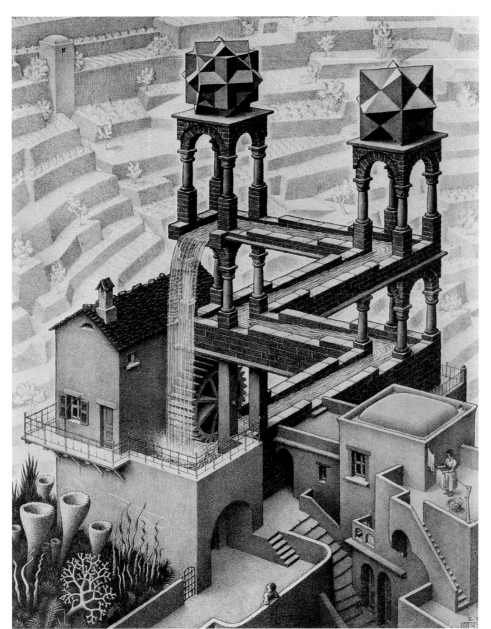

FIGURE **13-19**

Escher. *Waterfall.*

Lithograph, 1961. *(© 1996 M.C. Escher/Cordon Art—Baarn—Holland. All rights reserved.)*

FIGURE **13-20**
Illusions of length. **Left**, Müller-Lyon illusion. The two central lines appear of different length. **Right**, Top hat illusion. The hat appears taller than wide.

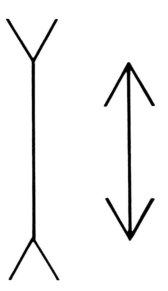
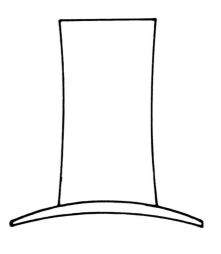

FIGURE **13-21**
Seurat. *The Clipper*.
1890. The sailboat appears taller than wide, but the dimensions are equal. *(The Solomon R. Guggenheim Museum, New York. Gift of Solomon R. Guggenheim June 28, 1937, Photograph by Robert E. Mates © The Solomon R. Guggenheim Foundation, New York [FN 37.718].)*

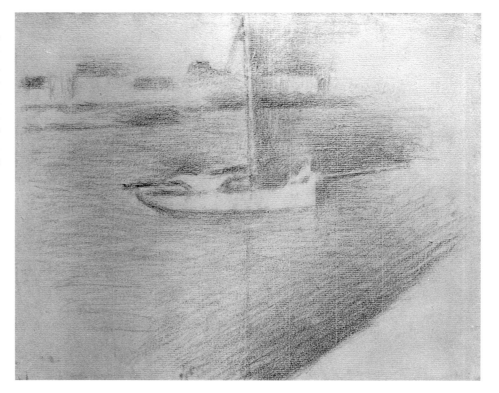

illusion, a line is misjudged to be short with arrowheads on either end or long with flaring terminal lines. The top hat appears much taller than wide, although the height and width are actually identical. Neural phenomena may play some role in the way comparisons of size are formulated in the brain, but it seems likely that these judgments are also conditioned by our expectations of relative size based on lifetime experience. These illusions appear in pictorial art, as they do in the world, whenever the subject matter meets the necessary conditions. For example, boats with masts usually appear taller than wide, although this may sometimes be illusory (Fig. 13-21).

mark in an Abstract-Expressionist painting."[11] In other words, the patterns of her art may have illusory content (or origins) but the final expression of her paintings are a result of independent experimentation and artistic judgment. This is exemplified in *Breathe*, which resembles one of the original diagrams (Fig. 13-22) that Mach used to illustrate perceptual effects of contrast.[12] In Riley's transmutation (Fig. 13-23), the pattern takes on a life of its own and no longer evokes Mach bands.

A contradictory opinion of op art has been expressed by an eminent neuroscientist, T. Shipley, who wrote: "For the scientist, 'Op' art is old hat and yet tremendous fun. . . . The eye performs as water runs down the hill. But 'Op' art is true, generally, in a pig's eye, and *moiré* [an optical pattern] can be seen perfectly by the camera. Indeed all this art is visual, hence optical, simply because the mind is irrelevant. But it is in the mind that the ends of science and of art meet. . . . Not much else can be said of a merely peripheral art; it falls horrendously short of its goal."[13] Perhaps Shipley should read more Riley as well as look at her art. To call op art a mere perceptual game is to miss the essential point of art. The question is not whether an Escher is equivalent to Rembrandt, or Vasarely to Monet, but

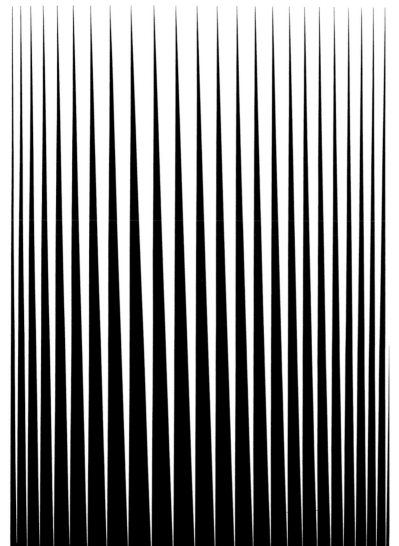

FIGURE 13-23

Riley. *Breathe*.

Emulsion on canvas, 1966. The wedges in this design, in comparison with those of Fig. 13-22, are of larger size and narrow continuously. There is no Mach band effect. The actual painting is of an entirely different scale, being nearly 10 feet by 7 feet in size. (*Museum Boymans-van Beuningen, Rotterdam.*)

whether any or all of these artists created new sensations, pleasures, and ideas. Understanding the scientific basis of vision, and the hardwired or softwired nature of illusions, should not diminish the appreciation of optical art; if anything, it allows the viewer to appreciate better how the artist has built on these illusory phenomena (which are common to all of us) to create additional effects that are special to human experience.

Riley's *Descending* (see Fig. 13-4) is a case in point. For me, it creates a sense of tension and instability that is quite powerful and quite unique. The shimmer in the picture comes from the physiologic observation that our eyes are continuously in motion, but Riley's painting also imposes a sense of urgency beyond the shimmer, which comes from the illusory curving lines and the conflict we feel between the pattern and its potential three dimensionality. These mixed sensations are not optical alone; they do involve the mind and they do represent art.

It is hard to leave the subject of illusion without considering at least briefly the subject of surrealism. In surrealism, illusion is used not so much for its visual effects but for its intellectual effects. When Magritte (Fig. 13-24) shows fragments of a scene upon the broken panes of a window, he is not only creating a visual illusion (in the sense that you are not sure what is painting and what is real), but he is also asking you to ponder on that very dilemma (which is not so far from Plato's question about whether any representation can in fact be reality). Yves Tanguy painted strange landscapes filled with objects that tantalize our senses as if we should somehow recognize them. The power of these images comes from our expectation of what we think we should see, as much as from our recognition of what we do see. The illusions of surrealism lie in the realm of softwiring

FIGURE **13-24**

Magritte. *The Key of the Fields.*

Oil, 1936. (Thyssen-Bornemisza Museum, Madrid, Spain. © Copyright 1996 C. Herscovici, Brussels/Artists Rights Society [ARS], New York. Nimatallah/Art Resource, NY.)

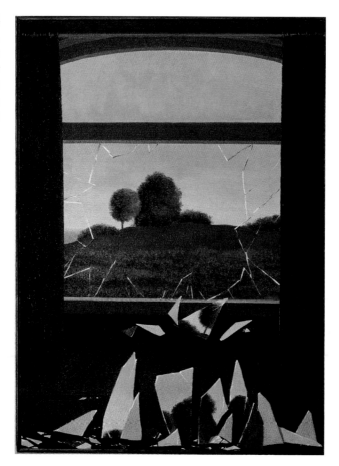

because they are intended for our mind as much as our eye. Like optical artists, the surrealists have at times been criticized as "nonartists," because their paintings are a means to an intellectual end, for which the artistic expression sometimes seem secondary. Personally, I find these arguments rather irrelevant, because the eye and the intellect cannot be separated in any artistic endeavor. The melted clocks of Dali are disturbing in large measure because of the stark and pseudorealistic landscapes in which Dali has artistically placed them. We view Asian art in terms of beauty, but many Asians will view it in terms of content. The glorious triptychs of Byzantine art were designed to teach the catechism to the masses, but beauty was important also to catch the eye of the audience.

This chapter has emphasized that some aspects of illusory sensation have a physical origin within retinal or visual cortical circuitry, while others depend on cultural bias or past visual experience. However, as Riley has pointed out, "Everyone knows by now, that neuro-physiological and psychologic responses are inseparable."[11] Psychology itself has a neural basis, and no hardwired illusion is free from psychologic overlay. Furthermore, few illusions fall purely or totally within either category. Part of the problem is that the very concept of illusion is in some respects illusory. Mach pointed out over 100 years ago that "the expression 'sense-illusion' shows that we have not yet become conscious of the fact that the senses neither falsely nor correctly manifest external events. . . . The only exact thing we can say about the sense organs is that under different circumstances they produce different sensations and perceptions."[14] Illusions are but one fact of biologic and psychologic visual processing, and as such they are but one tool (and one constraint) among many that contribute to the construction and appreciation of art.

— REFERENCES —

1. Rock I: *Perception*, Scientific American Library, New York, 1984.
2. Arnheim R: *Art and Visual Perception*, University of California Press, Berkeley, 1974.
3. Gombrich EH: *Art and Illusion*, Princeton University Press, Princeton, N.J., 1969.
4. Zeki S, Lamb M: The neurology of kinetic art, *Brain* 117:607-636, 1994.
5. Rushton WAH: King Charles II and the blind spot, *Vision Res* 19:225, 1979; Southall JPC: note 4, in H. von Helmholtz: *Treatise on Physiological Optics*, vol 2, Optical Society of America, 1924, p. 29.
6. Richards W: Obituary: H.-L. Teuber, *Vision Res* 18:357-359, 1978.
7. Lashley KS: Patterns of cerebral integration indicated by the scotomas of migraine, *Arch Neurol Psychiat* 46:331-339, 1941.
8. Kuffler SW, Nicholls JG, Martin AR: *From Neuron to Brain*, 2 ed, Sinauer Associates, Sunderland, Mass., 1984, pp. 58-59.
9. Penrose LS and Penrose R: Impossible objects: A special type of visual illusion, *Br J Psychol* 49:31-33, 1958.
10. Gombrich,[3] pp. 210-211.
11. Riley B: Perception is the medium, *Art News* 64:32-33, 66, 1965.
12. Mach E: Über die Wirkung der räumlichen Vertheilung des Lichtreizes auf die Netzhaut, *Sitz d Wiener Akad d Wissen* 52:303-322, 1866.
13. Shipley T: Editorial: The "Op" in modern art, *Vision Res* 6:1-2, 1966.
14. Mach E: On the dependence of retinal points on one another. Translated and reprinted in F Ratliff: *Mach Bands: Quantitative Studies on Neural Networks in the Retina*, Holden-Day, San Francisco, 1965, pp. 307-320.

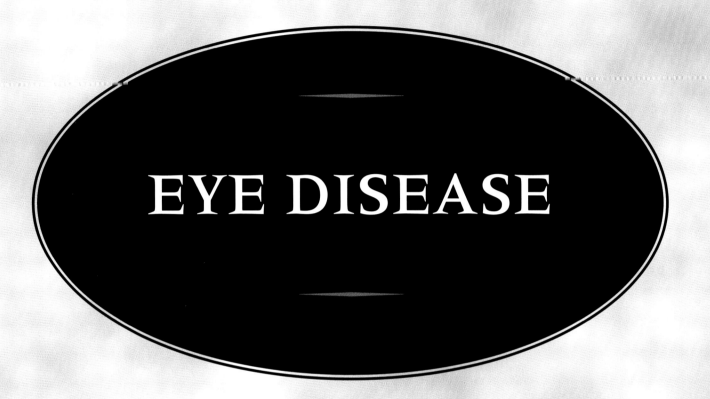

Part Six

EYE DISEASE

Chapter Fourteen

ARTISTIC VISION IN OLD AGE

CLAUDE MONET

James G. Ravin

Claude Monet (1840-1926) was the quintessential Impressionist. His 1873 painting *Impressionism: Sunrise* gave Impressionism its name. He lived to the ripe old age of 86 and died in 1926. This was well past the years of French Impressionism, for the eight Impressionist shows were held from 1874 to 1886. There is a distinct difference between his paintings of the 1870s and 1880s and his works created from World War I to the end of his life. The changes occurred slowly, but there can be no mistaking the late paintings, done with very broad strokes of the brush in bright colors. Monet's cataracts are known to have been present by 1912. There certainly is a temporal correlation of his cataract problem and his changes in style. Many of the late paintings depict the world in broad swirls and slashes of color. Seen up close the forms disappear. For this reason the late paintings of Monet are often considered a link to artistic movements that followed, particularly Abstract Expressionism. The paintings of Pollock and de Kooning seem now to be part of a natural evolution from the late canvases of Monet.

TRANSITIONS AFTER REACHING THE AGE OF FIFTY

By 1890 Monet had lived half a century. He had been working toward the ambitious goal of creating several paintings in series, which presented the same subject under a variety of light and atmospheric conditions and at different times of the day. This was a more focused and systematic version of his earlier Impressionist work. He would move from canvas to canvas as lighting conditions changed. The series paintings include some of his best known themes: grain-stacks, poplars, and Rouen Cathedral.

Except for the normal effects of aging, in 1890 Monet's eyes were not yet giving him the problems he was to develop during the first decade of the twentieth century. The difficulties he encountered in painting were not ocular. Instead, he was struggling with the problem of motivation. In July 1890 he wrote, "I am feeling very low and profoundly disgusted with painting. It is nothing but constant torture! Don't expect to see any new works; the little I have managed to do is destroyed, scraped off, or staved in."[1]

A few years later, as he approached the age of 60 (Fig. 14-1), Monet reminisced: "What I do know is, that life with me has been a hard struggle, not for myself alone, but for my friends as well. And the longer I live and the more I realize how difficult a thing painting is, and in one's defeat he must patiently strive

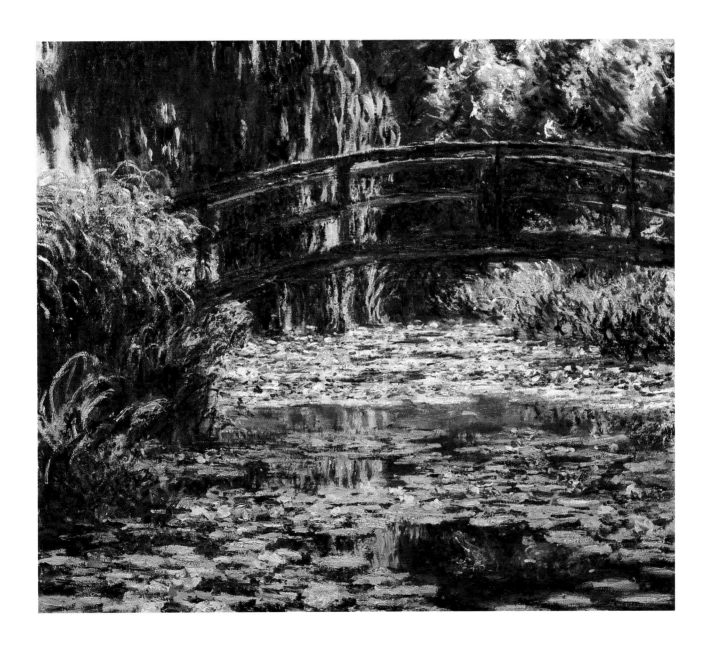

on."[2] Self-confidence was never Monet's long suit. Fortunately, he was able to rely on family and friends for support. His wife, Alice, his step-daughter Blanche (who was also his daughter-in-law), and his close friend, the French statesman Georges Clemenceau, were reliable props for this artist as he aged.

Monet's eyesight become a problem early in the new century. He was aware of his diminished vision by 1908. During a painting expedition to Venice in that year, Monet encountered difficulty handling colors, but he felt that his ability to handle forms was not impaired. He may have relied on others in choosing tints, for the problem of color is not easily noted in looking at the canvases he produced at that time. His depiction of space and depth in some of the Venetian scenes is not particularly skillful. Monet was not pleased with many of the works he had created, and he destroyed several of them. An article about Monet, published in 1908, described his difficulties in sad terms: "Partly because of overstrain, partly because of dissatisfaction, M. Monet became extremely irritable and morose, and at last actually cut a few of his canvases to shreds."[3]

Monet could be temperamental. An American painter wrote, "His opinion of his own work was not, however, always calmly judicial. On one occasion, particularly disgusted at his own inadequacy, he decided to give up painting altogether. He was painting from his boat at the time, so overboard flew the forevermore useless paint box, palette, brushes and so forth into the peaceful waters of the little Epte."[4]

THE CATARACT PROBLEM

By 1912 Monet was having a great deal of difficulty with his eyesight. His doctor in the countryside, Jean Rebiere, M.D., diagnosed bilateral cataracts. Monet consulted several ophthalmologists in Paris. One, A. Polack, M.D., must have been very sympathetic to Monet's plight, since he was an artist as well as a physician. Polack came to Paris in 1892 to study painting at the Ecole des Beaux-Arts. He transferred to the medical school of Paris, where he wrote his doctoral thesis on the effect of the refractive status of artists' eyes on their education and work. He became a professor of physiologic optics at the Institute d'Optique, was a scientist at the Centre National de la Recherche Scientifique, and director of the section of optics at the Laboratoire Scientifique du Louvre.[5] Polack confirmed the diagnosis of Monet's cataracts but advised that surgery be deferred.[6]

Monet consulted a second eminent ophthalmologist, A. Valude, M.D. Valude was an expert in cataract surgery and had given an important presentation on this topic at an international congress of ophthalmology a few years earlier. He was the author of a textbook of ophthalmology and coeditor of the *Encyclopedie francaise d'ophtalmologie*. He was a founding member of the Ophthalmological Society of Paris and an owner of the journal *Annales d'oculistique*.[7] Valude's advice to Monet was basically the same as that given by Polack.[8] Monet was deathly afraid of surgery. He discussed his problem in depth with his friend Clemenceau, who was a physician as well as a politician. Clemenceau's father and paternal grandfather also were physicians. Following the examination by Valude, Clemenceau wrote Monet to reassure him that he was not in danger of becoming blind. However, Monet's right eye was useless visually, since the cataract was nearly mature. Clemenceau noted that the cataract in Monet's right eye could be operated on and that "continuation of vision is assured."[8] Monet, ever anxious, preferred to do nothing more than try some eyedrops prescribed by Valude.

Monet soon consulted a third ophthalmologist, Victor Morax, M.D., the "dean" of French ophthalmology. Morax was a productive research scientist with a laboratory at the Institut Pasteur, and was a coeditor of the *Annales d'oculistique*.

Morax was an excellent surgeon and an enthusiastic teacher.[7] He took care of Marie Curie when she developed cataracts. Morax was in favor of surgery for Monet, but the artist remained intensely afraid of any operation.

Monet was elated when he met in Paris a German ophthalmologist named Count Weiser. Weiser promised Monet a nonsurgical cure for cataracts if he would only come to Germany for treatment. However, the opinions Monet received about this doctor were so discouraging that he never took up the offer.[8]

Monet consulted a fifth ophthalmologist, Richard Liebreich, M.D., in 1913. The eminent Liebreich, at age 83, was too elderly to be a vigorous surgeon. He was an accomplished artist who had created the illustrations for his important *Atlas of Ophthalmoscopy* and had studied at the Ecole des Beaux-Arts in Paris. His article on the effect of eye disease on the artists Turner and Mulready had been published separately on both sides of the English Channel and had an enormous impact for decades. Edgar Degas was well aware of it (see Chapter 17). Liebreich described two changes in visual perception that occur with aging, which are due to changes in the lens of the eye. First, Liebreich noted that as the lens thickens with age, it can scatter light. Liebreich felt that this change had occurred with Turner. Second, as the lens thickens, it develops a yellowish discoloration, which prevents some colors from reaching the retina. Liebreich believed that the changes in the colored pigments used by the artist Mulready were due to this type of change in the lenses of his eyes. In 1913 Liebreich was ending an amazing career that had brought him to the highest ranks of medicine in three different countries. He had been a student under Helmholtz in Germany, when the latter made the earth-shattering invention of the ophthalmoscope, and had been the right hand man of von Graefe in Berlin. Von Graefe is considered to have been the greatest ophthalmologist to have ever lived. Liebreich reached the pinnacle of French ophthalmology when he cured the mother of the French Empress Eugenie of acute glaucoma through surgery. (This was prior to the discovery of local anesthesia.) When Napoleon III's empire crumbled in 1870, Liebreich traveled to England with the imperial family. He was named chair of ophthalmology at St. Thomas Hospital and medical school in London and ophthalmic surgeon to the hospital.[9] Monet also left France during the Franco-Prussian War, to avoid military service, and, like Liebreich, went to London. St. Thomas Hospital also links Monet and Liebreich. Many of the canvases Monet painted of the Thames and the Houses of Parliament were done from a room in that hospital. It is not known if they met before 1913, but certainly they had much in common. Liebreich examined Monet and found the artist had no useful vision with his right eye. He prescribed glasses that had no power for the right eye. For the left eye, his prescription was −1.75 sphere for distance, indicating the artist was moderately nearsighted. For near sight, he prescribed +1.50 sphere.[10]

During the next few years, Monet refused to have anything done about his cataracts. He painted very little during the war years of 1914 to 1917. Finding a physician to care for civilians was not simple, since most were busy with the troops. Monet was very interested in the cataract problem of the American Impressionist who was living in France, Mary Cassatt (see Chapter 15). Her ophthalmologist was another American expatriate, Louis Borsch, M.D. Borsch cared for the ocular problems of the author James Joyce. Unfortunately, neither patient did well. Cassatt underwent cataract surgery to one eye in 1917 and to the other in 1919. The results were poor for both eyes, and Cassatt was forced to give up her artistic career. This may have been due to complications of her diabetes. It may also have been related to the radiation therapy she received to treat the diabetes. Her unfortunate surgical results did not encourage Monet to undergo the same procedure. He described his curiosity about Cassatt's vision in a letter to Clemenceau in November 1919. Aware she had just been operated on, he said he was going to find out about her condition and then make up his mind. He made up his mind to wait longer.

A reporter interviewed Monet in 1918. Monet described what had been happening to him during the last 5 years:

> I no longer perceived colors with the same intensity, I no longer painted light with the same accuracy. Reds appeared muddy to me, pinks insipid, and the intermediate or lower tones escaped me. As for forms, they always appeared clear and I rendered them with the same decision.
>
> At first I tried to be stubborn. How many times, near the little bridge where we are now, have I stayed for hours under the harshest sun sitting on my campstool, in the shade of my parasol, forcing myself to resume my interrupted task and recapture the freshness that had disappeared from my palette! Wasted efforts. What I painted was more and more dark, more and more like an "old picture," and when the attempt was over I compared it to former works, I would be seized by a frantic rage and slash all my canvases with my penknife.[11]

FIGURE   14-2

Monet. *Japanese Footbridge at Giverny.*

Oil on Canvas, c. 1923. *(Musée Marmottan, Paris. Copyright Musée Marmottan.)*

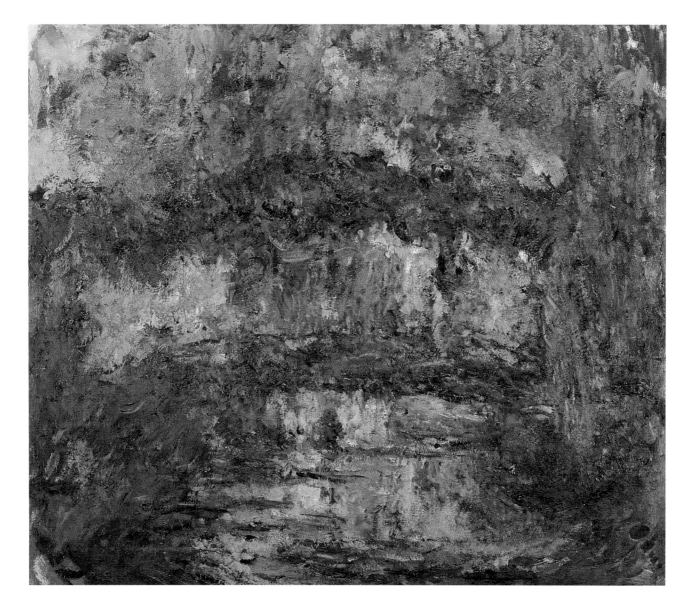

For a brief period he felt his visual problems had improved. Monet continued to have difficulties with subtle, delicate colors viewed up close. He felt he could see better when he stepped back a few feet. He began to paint once more. His attempts made him feel he could not paint in bright light conditions, and he had difficulty distinguishing between colors that were similar. He could still recognize vivid colors, especially if they were seen against a dark background. Since bright sunlight overwhelmed him, he stopped painting during the middle of the day. He realized that his choices of colors were poor and he destroyed many of his canvases. To avoid confusing pigments, he examined the labels on his tubes carefully and kept the paints on his palette in a regular, unvarying sequence in order to minimize errors.

His paintings of water lilies and weeping willows done between 1918 and 1922 show a loss of form. The yellow-brown cataracts through which he viewed the world filtered out violet and blue colors, as well as some of the greens. The paintings he made at that time included less of these colors and more yellows, reds, and browns (Fig. 14-2; see also Fig. 14-4).

In 1914 Clemenceau and a few other individuals encouraged Monet to donate a group of his water lily paintings to the government of France, as Monet's contribution to the war effort. Monet agreed and wrote Clemenceau on November 12, 1918: "Dear and great friend, I have stayed up late to finish two decorative panels that I would like to sign the day of victory, and I am going to ask you to act as intermediary to offer them to the country."[12]

A plan to donate 12 large canvases was announced officially in 1920. The next year, Monet tried to extricate himself from this obligation. He felt that he was incapable of completing the task. Clemenceau, unhappy, even angry with Monet, realized that failure to complete this project would be an embarrassment to himself and to the artist. He persuaded Monet to sign a notarized document in which Monet agreed formally to donate 19 panels to France. The government agreed to house them permanently in a small museum, the Orangerie des Tuileries, in the center of Paris, just off the Place de la Concorde.

Cézanne once quipped, "Monet is only an eye, but what an eye."[13] Clemenceau described how Monet's vision differed from his own:

> We do not see things in anything like the same manner. I open my eyes and I see forms, shades of color which I take, until disproved, for the passing aspect of things as they are. My eye stops at the reflecting surface and goes no deeper. With you, it is entirely different. The steel of your eyesight breaks the crust of appearances, and you penetrate the inner substance of things in order to decompose it into projectors of lights which you recompose with the brush, so that you may reestablish subtly upon our retinas the effect of sensations in their fullest intensity. And while I, looking at a tree, see nothing but a tree, you . . . , eyes half closed, think to yourself, "How many tones of how many colors are there in the gradations of light on this simple trunk?"[14]

Monet's eyes continued to give him difficulties. He described the problem he was having in complying with the terms of his agreement in a letter dated May 8, 1922: "I wished to profit from what little [remained of] my vision in order to bring certain of my decorations to completion. And I was gravely mistaken. For in the end I had to admit that I was ruining them, that I was no longer capable of making something of beauty. And I destroyed several of my panels. Today I am almost blind and I have to renounce work completely."[15]

Having outlived two wives and one of his two sons, Monet relied heavily on his friend Georges Clemenceau for support. Since Clemenceau was a physician, and he knew many members of the medical community, he had a strong influence on Monet when questions of health arose. At Clemenceau's urging, Monet consulted still another ophthalmologist in September 1922. This was Charles

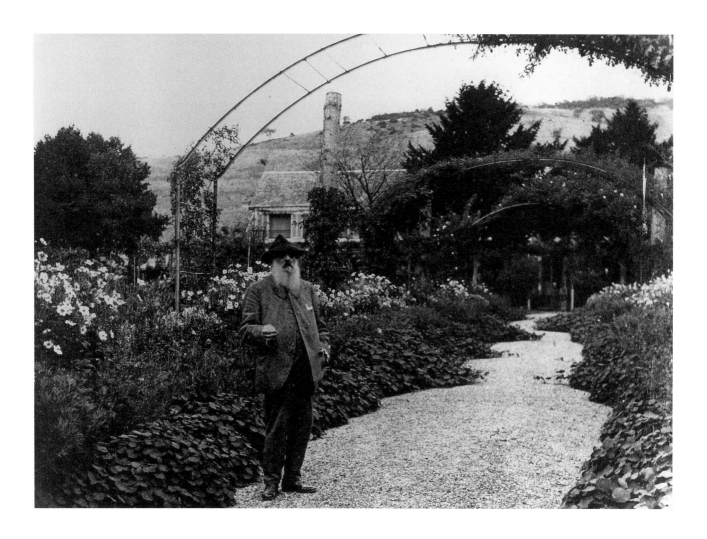

Coutela, M.D. Coutela was an accomplished surgeon, who was later honored by being named a Commander of the Legion of Honor and a member of the prestigious Academy of Medicine.[16]

In September 1922 Coutela found that Monet could only see light and the direction from which a light source was projected into his right eye. With the left eye Monet could read only 20/200. Monet was still psychologically unprepared for surgery. Coutela prescribed eyedrops to dilate the pupil of Monet's left eye, in the very optimistic hope that this might allow more rays of light to penetrate the cataractous lens of his left eye and reach the retina. The attempt was doomed to failure. The cataract was too dense.

Monet must have been extremely anxious that this experiment would succeed. Before a week was up, he wrote enthusiastically to Coutela: "It is all simply marvelous. I have not seen so well for a long time, so much so that I regret not having seen you sooner. The drops have permitted me to paint good things rather than the bad paintings which I had persisted in making when seeing nothing but fog."[17]

The effect was short lived, for Monet wrote Coutela again, in October 1922, to make plans for surgery to his right eye.[18] However, he could not convince himself to undergo an operation. In November he wrote Clemenceau of his apprehension and his nightmares and said he just was too tormented to have the surgery yet.[19] Clemenceau utilized all of his persuasive powers to convince Monet to have the operation. He continued to remind Monet of the agreement to finish the paintings for France.

SURGERY

Finally, in January 1923, Monet underwent a two-stage cataract operation to his right eye. A preliminary iridectomy was the first procedure. This was done at the Ambroise-Paré Clinic in Neuilly, a suburb of Paris. Later that month Coutela performed a second procedure, an extracapsular extraction of the cloudy lens.[20] Still extremely nervous, Monet was nauseated and vomited during the operation, to the consternation of his surgeon. Postoperatively, the 83-year-old patient (Fig. 14-3) was difficult to manage. He adapted poorly to the regimen of lying flat on his back for several days without a pillow. Sandbags were placed alongside his body to prevent any movement. All he was allowed to eat or drink was some bouillon and lime tea. Both eyes were bandaged shut. Saying he preferred to be blind rather than have his eyes covered, Monet tried to rip off the bandages. He was forcibly restrained from doing so. After discharge from the clinic, he returned home to Giverny. He was given a temporary pair of glasses to wear 3 weeks after surgery.

During the next few months, he developed a complication that caused him to undergo a third operation on the right eye. The posterior capsule of the lens became cloudy. Monet became depressed and refused to leave his bed. He wrote Coutela on June 22, 1923, saying,

> I am absolutely discouraged, and as much as I read, not without effort, fifteen to twenty pages per day, outdoors from a distance, I cannot see anything with or without glasses [with the right eye]. And for two days black spots [floaters] have bothered me.
>
> Remember that it has been six months since the first operation, five since I left the clinic, and four that I have been wearing glasses. It has taken me four or five weeks to get used to my new vision! Six months that I would have been able to work, if you had told me the truth. I would have been able to finish the *Decorations* that I was supposed to deliver in April and I am now uncertain if I will be able to finish them as I would have liked.
>
> It is to my great chagrin that I regret having had this fatal operation. Pardon me for speaking so frankly and let me tell you that it is criminal to have put me in this situation.[21]

Coutela responded quickly, reassuring Monet that this vision could be restored and convincing him to undergo the required procedure. Coutela described the events that followed:

> Afterwards as had been predicted, the inevitable thickening of the capsule occurred: This did not make me anxious, but caused a difficult time for Monet. He was desolated. The period which followed at Giverny was a time of profound discouragement and despair; he saw himself blind forever and, completely demoralized, refused to leave his bed. When the eye calmed down after the first operation I proceeded with the extraction of this contrary membrane. This operation, done at Giverny, in his home [on July 17, 1923], allowed him to obtain visual acuity of 7/10 [about 20/30] with the correction of +10.00 +4.00 × 90; I was reassured by the final result.[20]

THE POSTOPERATIVE PERIOD

The next step was to get Monet to adapt to cataract glasses. This was not an easy task. Monet had only one eye operated on and refused to have the second eye done. He could not use the two eyes together with his new glasses. The high-

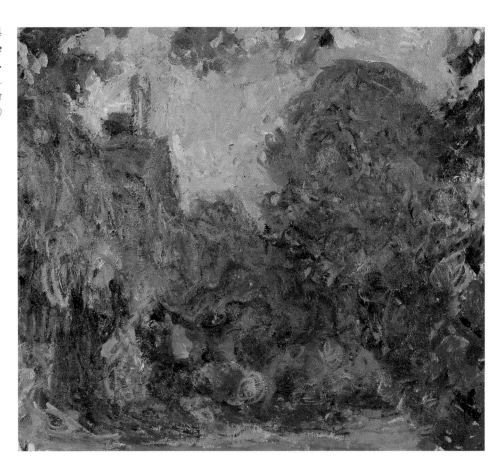

powered lens over his right eye prevented this. Since his left eye still contained a dense yellow-brown nuclear cataract, his color perception with the two eyes differed markedly. Violets and blues could simulate the retina of his right eye, while these colors could not penetrate the cataract in his left eye.[22] As an artist, he was acutely aware of these problems.

Figs. 14-4 and 14-5, although not dated precisely, may illustrate these differences in Monet's two eyes. Both depict his house as viewed from the same location in his garden, during the same season. They were sketches, possibly done with one eye at a time, to test his abilities in the postoperative period. The blue work would have been made using the operated right eye, and the yellow-brown canvas with the unoperated left eye.

Monet complained that objects curved abnormally with his new glasses and that colors were strange. Coutela was not so troubled. On August 21, 1923, he wrote Clemenceau: "His vision at near may be considered nearly perfect after correction. . . . For distant vision the result is less extraordinary: Mr. Monet has 3/10 to 4/10 vision [20/50 to 20/70], which is not bad, but he will require a little bit of training because the vision for distance is more or less restricted. In brief, I am very satisfied.[23] Monet wrote a sad letter to Coutela, August 27, 1923, describing the difficulties he was having with the glasses: "I have just received them today but I am absolutely desolated for, in spite of all my good will, I feel that if I take a step, I will fall on the ground. For near and far everything is deformed, doubled, and it has become intolerable to see. To persist seems dangerous to me."[24]

Three days later Monet wrote Clemenceau again: "To confirm what I said in my telegram after new trials with the lenses and with small doses, on Coutela's advice: I'm doing exercises and can read easily; that much is certain and it's restoring my confidence, but the distortion and exaggerated colours that I see are quite terrifying. As for going for a walk in these spectacles, it's out of the question for the moment anyway, and if I was condemned to see nature as I see it now, I'd prefer to be blind and keep my memories of the beauties I've always seen."[25] Clemenceau had wanted Monet to have both eyes operated on. Monet steadfastly refused. He stated his reasons in a letter to Clemenceau dated September 22, 1923:

> I have to say that in all sincerity and after much deliberation, I absolutely refuse (for the moment at least) to have the operation done to my left eye; you are far away and can have no idea of the state I'm in as regards my sight and the alteration of colours, and you cannot do anything to help me.
>
> I can see, read, and write and I fear that this is very probably the only result that can be obtained. So unless I find a painter, of whatever kind, who's had the operation and can tell me that he can see the same colours he did before, I won't allow it.
>
> I'm expecting Coutela tomorrow. I hope he'll change my lenses and we'll see if there's an improvement. I've been patient, and now you must be too.[26]

Clemenceau consoled Monet, and Monet took up his brushes again in order to complete the water lily series (Fig. 14-6). He continued to have difficulties, both psychological and visual, as is apparent in this letter to Coutela dated April 9, 1924: "For months I have worked with obstinacy, without achieving anything good. I am destroying everything that is mediocre. Is it my age? Is it defective vision? Both certainly, but vision particularly. You have given me back the sight of black on white, to read and write, and I cannot be too grateful for that, but I am certain that the vision of [this] painter . . . is lost, and all is for nothing.

I am telling you this confidentially. I hide it as much as possible, but I am terribly sad and discouraged. Life is a torture for me."[27]

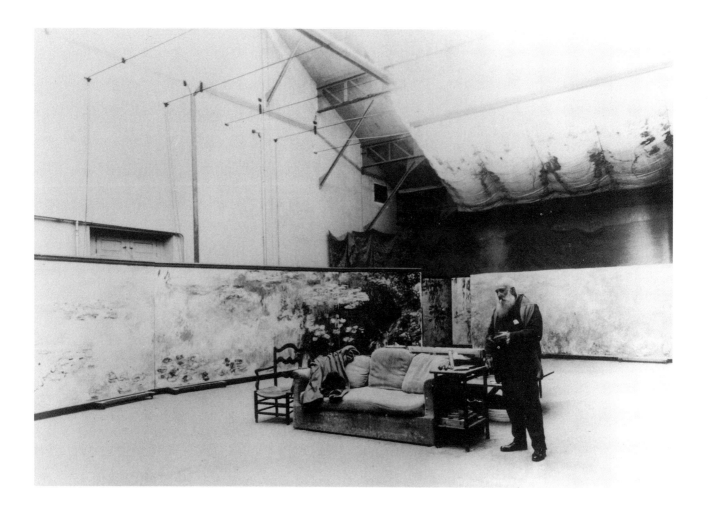

In the summer of 1924, still one more ophthalmologist was called in to care for the aging artist. This was Jacques Mawas, M.D., an esteemed researcher based at the Rothschild Eye Foundation.[28] He fit Monet with new lenses. Monet was easily discouraged and depressed. "At night I'm constantly haunted by what I'm trying to achieve. I get up exhausted every morning. The dawning day gives me back my courage. But my anxiety comes back too soon as I set foot in my studio. . . . Painting is so difficult. And a torture. Last fall I burned six canvases along with the dead leaves from my garden. It's hopeless. Still I wouldn't want to die before saying all that I have to say, or at least having tried to say it. And my days are numbered."[29]

Mawas worked long and hard with Monet. Monet described some of his difficulties to Mawas in March 1925:

I am quite late in giving you news concerning the outcome of my new glasses, but they arrived at such a bad period. I was very discouraged and I no longer hoped for better, so that I discontinued using these glasses which I probably might have accustomed myself to had they not completely disturbed me—eyesight trouble, the slightest color tones broken and exaggerated.

As soon as I am in a better frame of mind I will try to get used to them, though I am even more certain that a painter's eyesight can never be returned. When a singer loses his voice he retires; the painter who has undergone a cataract operation, must give up painting; and this is what I have been incapable of doing.[30]

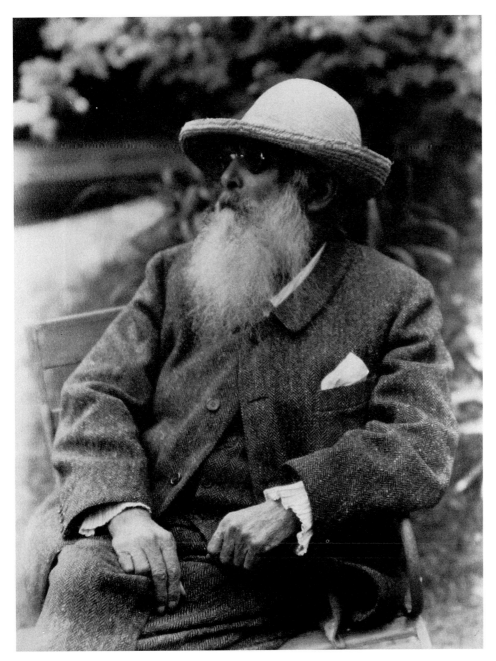

FIGURE 14-7

Monet in straw hat and glasses. Gelatin-silver print, c. 1926 by Nickolas Muray. *(The Museum of Modern Art, New York. Gift of Mrs. Nickolas Muray. Copyprint ©1996 The Museum of Modern Art, New York.)*

Monet's depressive mood improved by July 1925. "Since your last visit my vision is totally ameliorated. I am working harder than ever, am pleased with what I do, and if the new glasses are better still I would like to live to be one hundred."[31] His improved attitude was still present 10 days later in this letter to Dr. Coutela: "I am very happy to inform you that finally I have recovered by true vision and that nearly at a single stroke. In brief, I am happily seeing everything again and I am working with ardor."[32]

Monet painted almost to the day of his death in December 1926. The 86-year-old artist (Fig. 14-7) had been a chronic smoker, and he died of chronic obstructive pulmonary disease and cancer of the lung. A group of his water lily canvases was installed in the museum of the Orangerie in 1927, where they may be seen today. These paintings are the triumphs of an aged artist.

— **REFERENCES** —

1. Geffroy G: Monet: Sa vie, son oeuvre. Quoted in CF Stuckey (ed): *Monet, a Retrospective*, HL Levin, NY, 1985, p. 156.
2. Fuller WH: Claude Monet and his paintings. Quoted in Stuckey (ed),[1] p. 203.
3. Anonymous: The conscientious artist, *The Standard*, May 20, 1908. Quoted in Stuckey (ed),[1] p. 251.
4. Perry LC: Reminiscences of Claude Monet from 1889 to 1909, *American Magazine of Art*, March 1927. Quoted in Stuckey (ed),[1] p. 181.
5. Anonymous: Necrologie A. Polack, *Bulletins et Mémoires, Société Française d'Ophtalmologie*, 66:xci-xcii, 1953.
6. Wildenstein D: *Claude Monet Biographie et Catalogue Raisonne*, Lausanne et Paris, Bibliothèque des Arts, vol 4, 108, 1985.
7. Blodi FC: *Hirschberg's History of Ophthalmology*, vol IIC, Wayenbourg, Bonn, 1986, p. 643.
8. Wildenstein,[6] 4:77.
9. Ravin JG, Kenyon C: From von Graefe's clinic to the Ecole des Beaux-Arts. The meteoric career of Richard Liebreich, *Surv Ophthalmol* 37:221-228, 1992.
10. Wildenstein,[6] 4:108.
11. Thiebault-Sisson F: Les nympheas de Claude Monet à l'Orangerie des Tuileries, *La Revue de l'Art Ancien et Moderne* 52:45-46, 1927.
12. Monet C: Letter to Clemenceau dated November 12, 1918, Hoog M (ed): *Georges Clemenceau à son Ami Claude Monet*, Réunion des Musées Nationaux, Paris, 1993, p. 63.
13. Vollard A: *Paul Cézanne, His Life and Art*, Frank-Maurice, New York, 1926, p. 74.
14. Clemenceau G: *Claude Monet, The Winter Lilies*. Doubleday, Doran, Garden City, NY, 1930, pp. 18-19.
15. Stuckey CF: Blossoms and blunders: Monet and the state, II, *Art in America* 68:116, 1979.
16. Offret G: Necrologie, Charles Coutela, 1876-1969, *Arch d'Ophthalmol* 29:589-592, 1969.
17. Monet C: Letter to Coutela dated September 13, 1922, French Ophthalmologic Society, Paris.
18. Monet C: Letter to Coutela dated October 20, 1922, French Ophthalmologic Society, Paris.
19. Monet C: Letter to Clemenceau dated November 9, 1922, French Ophthalmologic Society, Paris.
20. Dittere M: Comment Monet recouvra la vue après l'opération de la cataracte, *Sandorama* 32:30, 1973.
21. Monet C: Letter to Coutela dated June 22, 1923, French Ophthalmologic Society, Paris.
22. Ravin JG: Monet's cataracts, *JAMA* 254:394-399, 1985.
23. Coutela C: Letter to Clemenceau dated August 21, 1923, French Ophthalmologic Society, Paris.
24. Monet C: Letter to Coutela dated August 27, 1923, French Ophthalmologic Society, Paris.
25. Monet C: Letter to Clemenceau dated August 30, 1923. In Wildenstein,[6] 5:416.
26. Monet C: Letter to Clemenceau dated September 23, 1923. In Wildenstein,[6] 5:416.
27. Monet C: Letter to Coutela dated April 9, 1924, French Ophthalmologic Society, Paris.
28. Dubois-Poulsen A: Jacques Mawas 1885-1976, *Ann d'Ocul* 209:325-331, 1976.
29. Delange R, Gordon R, Forge A: *Monet*, Abrams, New York, 1983, p. 247.
30. Monet C: Letter to Coutela dated March 25, 1925, French Ophthalmologic Society, Paris.
31. Hoschede DJ: *Claude Monet ce Mal Connu*, Cailler, Geneva, Switzerland, 1960, pp. 150-151.
32. Monet C: Letter to Coutela dated July 27, 1925, French Ophthalmologic Society, Paris.

CATARACTS, DIABETES, AND RADIUM

THE CASE OF CASSATT

James G. Ravin

Mary Cassatt (1844-1926) has often been considered the most famous American artist working during the last 100 years. Her main rivals for this honor are Whistler and Sargent. She is not as well known as she deserves to be. Her accomplishments were amazing for a nineteenth-century woman, since women were still expected to remain in the home and be occupied with household duties. Upon hearing of his daughter's plan to study in Europe, Cassatt's father exclaimed, "I would almost rather see you dead."[1] She studied at the Pennsylvania Academy of the Fine Arts for 4 years and then traveled across the Atlantic to study the works of the old masters in Europe. Finding the artistic environment in France especially encouraging, she spent most of the rest of her life there. By the age of 24 she had achieved success in the French academic art world. She exhibited works at the Salon several times. At that time, acceptance by the Salon, and not by private dealers, was the key to artistic success. However, she found that demands for conformity made by the juries for the Salon stifled her artistic development. She became friendly with several of the Impressionists, Degas in particular. She exhibited at four of the eight Impressionist shows and was the only American artist ever to exhibit with the Impressionists.

Cassatt is classified as an Impressionist, but her work differs from Impressionists such as Monet in several ways. Her characteristic themes were indoor scenes of mothers and children, rather than outdoor landscapes. Until

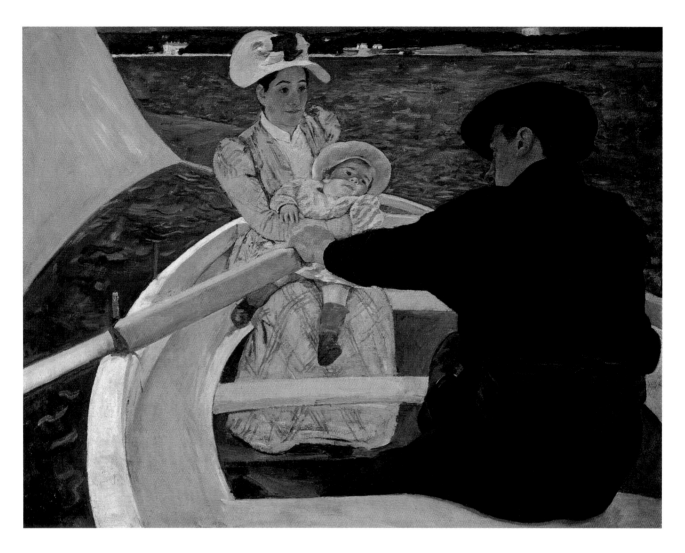

poor vision became a severe problem for her, her paintings were carefully composed (Fig. 15-1) and lacked the broken brush strokes typical of Monet and Pissarro. Her closest friend among the Impressionists was the witty and sarcastic Degas, who said of her, "I am not willing to admit that a woman can draw that well."[2]

She achieved recognition early in Europe but remained relatively unknown in America. Eventually she was recognized as a significant figure at home, but this was many years later. When she returned to Philadelphia in 1898, after having spent several decades in France, a local newspaper carried this casual note on the society page: "Mary Cassatt, sister of Mr. Cassatt, president of the Pennsylvania Railroad, returned from Europe yesterday. She has been studying painting in France, and owns the smallest Pekingese dog in the world."[3]

Cassatt was born in 1844, in what is now Pittsburgh, and died in 1926 at the age of 81 at her chateau in northern France. Visual problems began for her after 1900. Cataracts were diagnosed by 1912 when she was 68 years of age. In 1913 she was examined by Edmond Landolt, M.D., the famous French ophthalmologist, who also cared for Degas. Unfortunately, his records have not survived. By 1915, in the early years of World War I, she had to stop her art work altogether due to poor vision. Because it was wartime, it was difficult to find a doctor available to treat civilians. Her late paintings (Fig. 15-2) had become strident, harsh in color. The smooth texture of her earlier works was gone, replaced by a coarse type of painting that lacked any delicacy of touch. In 1917 she had cataract

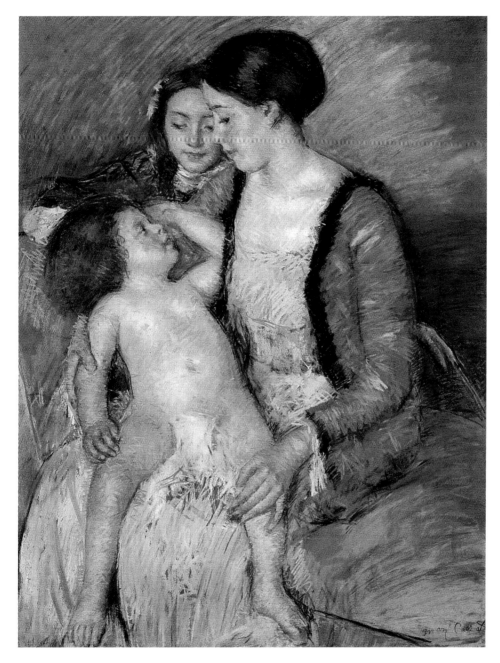

FIGURE   15-2

Cassatt. *Mother, Young Daughter, and Son.*

Pastel on paper, 1913. *(Memorial Art Gallery of the University of Rochester. Marion Stratton Gould Fund.)*

surgery performed on her right eye by Louis Borsch, M.D., an American oph-thalmologist who was married to a French woman. An opacity of the posterior lens capsule followed. In 1919 the left cataract was operated, but the result was poor. She could not read. As she continued to age, other medical problems became serious afflictions. Diabetes was diagnosed, and she was placed on a strict medical program to treat this disease.

Cassatt's letters give us important information about the health of her eyes. The largest collection of her correspondence is owned by the National Gallery in Washington, D.C. Significant passages in these letters concern her vision.

On July 16, 1913, she wrote, "My eyes have been greatly changed, my sight disturbed by incessant motoring in the south. . . . My eyes which have always been my strong point, are troubling me. If only I was sure of a good oculist, but Dr. Whitman is again away. I don't know for how long."[4]

A letter dated November 4, (1913?) said:

> It is dark and rainy, my oculist has turned out terribly. I have conjunctivi-
> tis, an inflammation of the eyelids. He said it was nothing, that I had good
> sight, one eye very good, the other not so good, but not very bad. Then when
> I saw him again, change of front. Wants to keep me here two months and try
> experiments on the poorer eye, trained nurse to assist at the operation twice
> a week! Dr. Whitman was horrified. He told me plainly it was to make
> money. My dear, it is hard that one goes for a little simple advice and to be
> tested for glasses and they (he is like most) sees a chance of making money
> and does not hesitate to rush making you blind! My theory is that they get
> so hardened with vivisection that human suffering is nothing to them.[4]

In a telegram dated August 21, 1915, from Paris, she wrote, "Am here care of
oculist. Must not read or write."[4] Another telegram, dated September 8, 1915,
says, "Sick eyes. Iritis with adhesion under treatment. Famous ophthalmologist if
he succeeds. Operation to be necessary. Love."[4]

A letter not dated, but approximately July 1916, noted that "Dr. Borsch treating my eyes, which keeps up hope, he still maintains though that I shall see to
work, but I do not believe it."[4] On December 12, 1917, from Paris, she wrote, "I
shall be very lonely, and as my sight gets dimmer every day, the operated eye will
not help my sight much, even though the secondary cataract is absorbed altogether which is very doubtful, if not almost quite sure."[4]

A letter dated December 28, 1917, read, "I am nearer despair than I ever was.
Operating on my right eye before the cataract was ripe is the last drop. I asked
Borsch if it was ripe and he assured me that it was! The sight of that eye is inferior but still I saw a good deal in spite of the cataract. Now I see scarcely at all."[4]
Cassatt's comments about ripeness imply that Borsch did an extracapsular procedure on the right eye, leaving the posterior capsule behind. The capsule would
nearly always opacify later, creating the need for a second operation to open the
cloudy capsule.

The following year, on July 13, 1918, Cassatt wrote: "The secondary cataract is
covering the right eye which was operated in October, and no doubt it can be
removed in the fall. The operation which was made in October and was followed
by so long a treatment was a complete failure and ought not to have been
attempted, if only it has not injured what there was of sight in that eye! The
cataract over the left eye, which is the eye in which depends my hope of future
sight, is not nearly ripe or I could not write you this. I do not believe it will be
ripe this year. . . . I could have gone up to see my oculist, but it would not have
served me for my eyes are not ready. . . . Dr. Borsch is oculist at the Grand Palais
and is in the French Army."[4]

In the following month, August 24, 1918, she wrote, "My sight is getting dimmer every day. I find writing tires my eyes. I look forward with horror to utter
darkness and then an operation which may end in as great a failure as the last
one."[4]

On May 24, 1919, she wrote that "the secondary cataract is to be opened and
that means two or three days in bed. The sugar and arterial pressure have been
diminished and the operation can be done, but there is not the slightest assurance
that the result will produce a return of sight in that eye. . . . I am to have the secondary cataract opened this week."[4]

Six months later, November 14, 1919, she wrote, "The operation was done on
October 22. . . . The operation was a very daring one as the cataract was not ripe
but he staked his reputation on the result. He is the only man in Paris capable of
doing such an operation and I am told few anywhere in the U.S. . . . I must only

write a little with one eye as I did before as the cotton is over the other still, and I must not use the other much."[4] Since surgery was to be undertaken while the cataract was not "ripe," Borsch probably employed the newer technique of intra-capsular extraction. But it is hard to believe that Borsch was the only ophthalmic surgeon in Paris capable of doing this.

The operation did not produce the desired result, for on March 28, 1920, she wrote, "I am old and so blind that I don't feel up to much. . . . I see less with the eye that was operated in October than I did with the one with a secondary cataract in it! Borsch knew that would be so and spoke of a film that sometimes formed after an operation for cataract even when the operation was ripe and that it was nothing to make a slit and then one saw! Which means of course another operation which equally I must submit to. I think the state of my eyes will I hope shorten my life. . . . My dear I can see no one, no pictures, no photos."[4] Two months later, on May 18, 1920, she wrote of the need for further surgery: "A secondary cataract is to be opened tomorrow."[4]

In 1921 Cassatt wrote: "Last May I had an operation upon my best eye. The operation was very successful and the oculist promised me I should paint again, but a hidden abscess in an apparently sound tooth caused a violent inflammation, and I have not yet recovered from it. Nor has the sight of the eye returned."[5] The theory of "focal infection" was popular at the time. Certainly infection in the teeth, or elsewhere, can spread to the eye. This was more common in the preantibiotic era than today and provided a convenient scapegoat when surgical results were suboptimal.

Also in 1921, she wrote, "I have had a very serious operation for cataract several weeks ago, and have my eye still bandaged, and can see very indifferently with the other eye which is my poor eye. I shall not be able to use my eyes, nor be allowed glasses for several months to come, after that my oculist promises great results. I do not allow myself such sanguine hopes."[5]

Other health matters, particularly diabetes, were of great importance to her. Prior to this series of letters about her eye problems, she described her treatment for diabetes. In a letter dated December 14, 1911, she wrote, "I am at the doctor's taking inhalations of radium. This is the eighth day, and I am suffering very much, which it seems would prove that it is doing me good, that it will be a success, provided I can stand it."[6]

Many forms of therapy were used to treat diabetes early in this century that appear bizarre today. It was not until 1920 that Banting et al. described their work with insulin, and they published their classic article about insulin in 1922.[7] Radiation therapy was tried for many diseases, including a number of ocular diseases. Considered in the context of that era, this new form of therapy was exciting and was used even to treat cataracts. It is not known if Cassatt's cataracts were treated by radiation, but two articles dating from this period are most interesting. Franklin and Cordes, successive chairmen of the department of ophthalmology at the University of California in San Francisco, published an article entitled "Radium for Cataract," in 1920 in the *American Journal of Ophthalmology*. They reported that "of the 31 patients under observation, 84.3% showed a change for the better. In the cases that showed a marked improvement, the opacities were very definitely thinned out; one of these, a very early nuclear cataract, disappeared entirely leaving no trace of the opacities. Radium is of proven value in the treatment of incipient cataracts."[8]

Similar statements were published in the radiologic literature. In 1920 an article in the *American Journal of Roentgenology* entitled "The Technic of Radium Application in Cataracts" concluded that "the application of radium is harmless to the normal tissues of the eye."[9] In the early days of radiation therapy, the dangers of radiation were not known. Many workers suffered severe complications, even

Marie Curie. Curie developed cataracts and had surgery done to each eye. Victor Morax. M.D., one of the ophthalmologists that treated Monet, took care of her.

As Cassatt's cataracts advanced, she became unable to paint in the finely detailed manner of her previous years (compare Fig. 15-1 with Fig. 15-2). She found working with pastel did not require the sharp acuity that oil painting had previously. Cassatt's close friend Degas worked more with pastels than oil paints when his vision diminished from what was probably macular degeneration. He lost the central vision in each eye. Each artist's late pastels were done in broad strokes on large pieces of paper. Their colors became limited in range with less gradation of the hue and were often strident. Details also diminished in the late works, for both artists were unable to create the delicacy of earlier paintings.

Deeply embittered, depressed, and disappointed by her visual problems, Cassatt stopped her artistic work after 1915. By 1918 she could not read. The vision loss shortened her artistic career by a dozen years. She died in 1926 at the age of 81, the same year in which Monet died.

Cassatt was surely a remarkable individual. In an era when most women stayed close to home, she traveled across the Atlantic to earn fame in Europe. Cassatt took an old theme, that of mother and child, and invigorated it with her own charm. She produced many touching works that fortunately do not come across as artificial or sentimental. Degas said of her work, "That is genuine. There is one who does as I do."[10] Her art is appealing to our taste today, with its combination of precise drawing, forms simplified by an Oriental influence and the bright colors of Impressionism.

— **REFERENCES** —

1. Hale N: *Mary Cassatt*, Doubleday, Garden City, N.Y., 1975, p. 31.
2. Hale,[1] p. 193.
3. Sweet FA: *Miss Mary Cassatt, Impressionist from Pennsylvania*, University of Oklahoma Press, Norman, 1966, p. 150.
4. Cassatt quotations are from the Cassatt correspondence in the National Gallery, Washington, D.C.
5. Sweet,[3] p. 198.
6. Hale,[1] p. 244.
7. Banting FG et al: Pancreatic extracts in the treatment of diabetes mellitus, *Can Med Assoc J* 12:141-146, 1922.
8. Franklin WS, Cordes FC: Radium for cataract, *Am J Ophthalmol* 3:643-647, 1920.
9. Levin I: The technic of radium application in cataracts, *Am J Roentgenol* 7:107-108, 1920.
10. Bullard EJ: *Mary Cassatt Oils and Pastels*, Watson-Guptill, New York, 1972, p. 13.

Chapter Sixteen

PISSARRO, THE TEARFUL IMPRESSIONIST

James G. Ravin

Camille Pissarro (1830-1903), the elder statesman of French Impressionism (Fig. 16-1), had a long artistic career. He was, with Claude Monet, a founder and leader of the French Impressionist movement. He was also a colleague and friend of Degas, Renoir, Seurat, Cassatt, and van Gogh. Pissarro was the only member of the Impressionist group to exhibit at every one of their shows, from 1874 until 1876. His productivity during the last 15 years of his life was hampered by recurrent infections around his right eye. These problems troubled him greatly and necessitated multiple visits to his ophthalmologist in Paris for care. When Pissarro was able to work, the ocular problems influenced his method of painting.

The history of Pissarro's malady is interesting for the light it sheds on a major artist's method of adjusting to adversity. The story also provides a view of one aspect of the history of medical care in the late nineteenth century, with interesting comparisons to medical care today. This artist was an ardent follower of homeopathic therapy. He acquired his mother's faith in homeopathy during a severe illness she had suffered many years earlier. Pissarro frequently consulted a book of remedies that he kept at home and often mailed advice to his children after they had grown and moved away.

Pissarro found an ophthalmologist who utilized homeopathic therapy in Daniel Parenteau, M.D. (1842-c. 1935). Parenteau was trained in traditional allopathic medicine but employed homeopathic medications. Although he advocated

FIGURE 16-1
Pissaro. Self-Portrait.
Oil on canvas, c. 1898. *(Dallas Museum of Art. The Wendy and Emery Reves Collection.)*

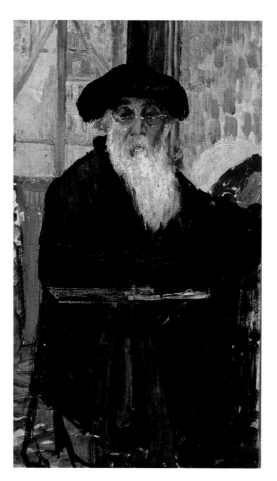

homeopathic drugs, he was not opposed to surgery. He was a member of the French Ophthalmologic Society[1] and of the Homeopathic Medical Society of France, and he was president of the latter society in 1901 and 1902.[2] Parenteau published occasionally in the homeopathic literature but more often in ophthalmologic medical publications. He wrote three books: *Leçons de Clinique Ophtalmologique*,[3] *Education de l'Oeil et son Hygiène*,[4] and *Thérapeutique Homéopathique en Ophtalmologie*.[5]

OCULAR PROBLEMS

Pissarro suffered from chronic infection of the tear sac with fistula formation during the last 15 years of his life. The date he first developed this is not known, but it certainly was present by 1889, when he described the results of a visit to his ophthalmologist. In May 1889 Parenteau found Pissarro's right nasal lacrimal duct was blocked. He probed the passages and found a bony obstruction. He told the artist that attempting to force a probe through the blocked area could create disastrous complications. Instead, he prescribed a homeopathic medication, Aurum, in the hope that it would allow the tissues around the bone to heal. He told Pissarro that healing would take at least 6 months and that he should take care to "avoid wind and dust, and wash the eye immediately with boric acid should anything get in it." Pissarro noted, "All that is hardly easy for a painter who ought to face the elements."[6]

Seven weeks later Pissarro reported that "Dr. Parenteau found that the lacrimal sac has flattened out but swelling persists near the lacrimal canal, at the inner corner of the eye. Because of this, I have to keep a dressing over my eye for at least a month. . . . If after a month things have not improved, it will be necessary to make a small incision in the swollen area to allow the tissues to heal properly, so that tears can flow normally."[7]

Nearly a year and a half later, in January 1891, Pissarro wrote his son Lucien, "I am very troubled at this moment. My eye has been irritated by the intense cold weather and is swollen. It is threatening to turn into an abscess. I must see Dr. Parenteau."[8] Later that month, he reported, "Parenteau has found me much better. . . . I must keep a bandage over the eye for ten more days. This is very annoying."[9] He continued, "I shall try to work with one eye. Degas does it and gets good results."[10]

In March 1891 Pissarro optimistically wrote Lucien, "My eye is going well. I saw Parenteau, who was very happy with the result. He advised me to put a patch over the eye in bad weather. In two weeks, if things are the same, if the walls of the tear sac come together, I will be cured. Things have gone well up till now. For a month I have not had any swelling."[11] But a month later he wrote, "A new abscess has developed. I am forced to suspend all work."[12] He returned to Paris and saw Parenteau, who probably drained the area again. Two days later Pissarro noted that the abscess was nearly gone.[13]

SECOND AND THIRD OPINIONS

Pissarro sought advice from other doctors. One young physician told him "destruction of the sac was not a good answer to his problem, since tears would continue to flow copiously." For a painter, this could be a serious difficulty that could prevent him from working. This doctor advised him "the only thing to do is to try to find the passage through bone into the nose." Pissarro met an older physician who told him "he had the same problem as I, and forty years earlier he had his first symptoms. This doctor's friends and colleagues advised surgery, but he declined, and the sac closed itself off. He lived that way for forty years without difficulty, except for a bit of tearing."[14] Pissarro then questioned Parenteau at greater length about these two alternatives, surgery versus medical therapy. At age 60, Pissarro was no longer young, and he was afraid of operative complications. He felt Parenteau had managed his case well and concluded he should continue with him.

TREATMENT IN THE LATE NINETEENTH CENTURY

Pissarro's consultants were aware of the level of understanding of lacrimal disease at the time. Lacrimal problems and their treatment had been described at length in the medical literature.[15,16]

Unfortunately for Pissarro, he never met the Italian surgeon Toti, who developed modern lacrimal surgery during Pissarro's lifetime. In 1904, the year following the artist's death, Toti published his method of dacryocystorhinostomy.[17]

Prior to the development of modern lacrimal surgery, two methods of treating dacryocystitis existed, removal of the sac and probing. Removal of the sac destroyed the pathway for tears to the nose and resulted in constant tearing.

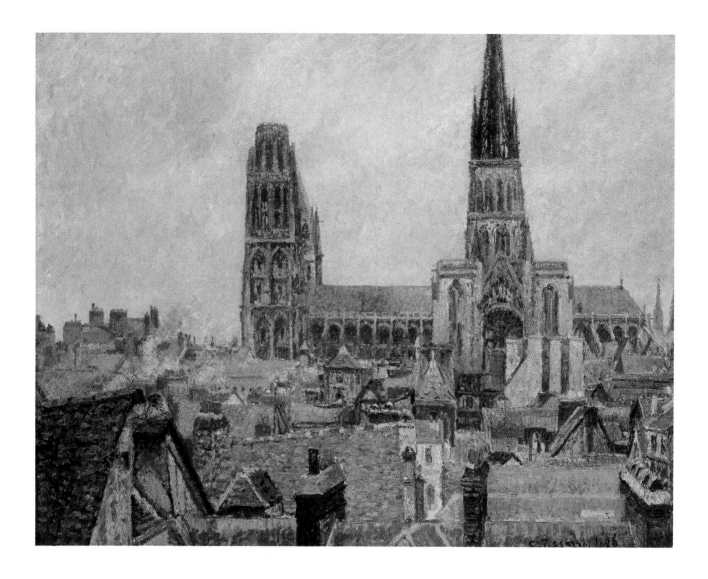

Probing the lacrimal drainage system often produced false passages, which could create cellulitis and further scarring.

On May 7, 1891, Pissarro wrote his son Lucien, "Parenteau has injected the area with silver nitrate, to close off the abnormal passageways. . . . I am getting used to the idea of having only one eye for working. This is much better than having none at all." A typical parent, Pissarro finished this letter to his son by giving him advice on taking care of himself. "You told me you have a bad cold. Take care of yourself. Do not neglect yourself, because so-called minor problems can become very serious. If you find that your nose is often blocked, see an eye doctor. If I had known Parenteau earlier, I would not have had my problem. The same thing can happen to you, considering the shape of your nose."[18]

PISSARRO'S PROBLEM SMOLDERED ALONG

Three months later, in July 1891, he wrote his son again. "I have really not had good luck, but I am being patient. . . . I am taking large doses of quinine as a preventive measure."[19]

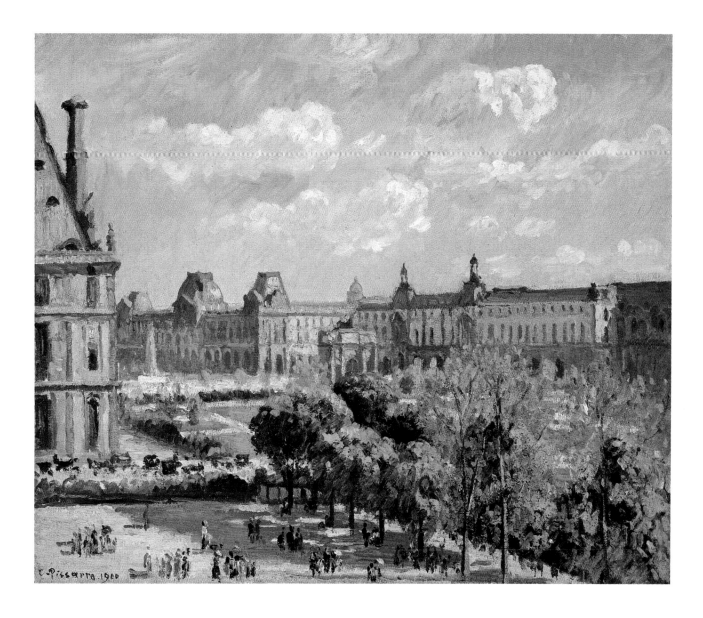

FIGURE   16-3

Pissarro. *La Place du Carrousel,*
Paris.

Oil on canvas, 1900. *(Ailsa Mellon*
Bruce Collection, © 1996 Board of
Trustees, National Gallery of Art,
Washington, D.C.)

During the next few years, the problem continued to smolder. He wrote Lucien in 1896: "Although an operation can cause unexpected complications, it should not be done if there is a chance of bony destruction, which there is not. . . . I am not nervous. What annoys me is to not be able to work outdoors."[20]

EFFECT ON HIS PAINTING

Pissarro adapted to the situation. Unable to work outdoors, he would paint indoors looking outward. His city-scapes of Rouen and Paris (Figs. 16-2 and 16-3), created over the next few years, were triumphs. In 1897 Pissarro began a letter to Lucien by prodding him, saying, "You ought to write me from time to time, to exercise your hand a little bit." He then described his ocular problem: "I am afraid of complications for my eye. I have gone daily for a dozen days to Parenteau, who has been cauterizing me and has been putting an astringent on the veins of the eye. . . . Parenteau gave me silver nitrate drops to put in the eye and on the lids.

This is hardly easy. Every morning there is more pus in the eye, so that I dare not venture a trip. Your mother advised me not to leave." Lucien was about to depart for London, to visit his brother, Titi, who was moribund from tuberculosis. Pissarro wrote, "I hope that you do not go, that you are busy with your work. Aren't you afraid that the London fog will be unfavorable for you? The weather has been exceptional here since you left. Now it is 3:30 and there is a beautiful golden sun outside with a slight mist."[21]

Lucien's brother Titi died 4 days later in November 1897 at age 24. Pissarro consoled Lucien. "I am happy to learn that you have been able to face the disastrous news of the death of our poor Titi, whom we loved so much, our hope, our pride. . . . But in such sad circumstances we must resign ourselves and think of those who are with us. . . . Finally, my dear Lucien, let's work to treat our wounds. I hope that you will be strong and that you will wrap yourself up, so to speak, in your art. . . . I must return to Parenteau, for cautery. I am improving, but I must persist."[22] Two years later in 1900, things had not changed: "The grippe has left me with inflammation of the eye. Parenteau is going to cauterize me."[23]

Shortly thereafter, Pissarro wrote: "I am much better thanks to the cauterization which I was able to undergo. The eye has returned to its normal state and there has been no pus since yesterday. Sadly, while I am not troubled by the eye, I have had severe pain in the kidneys, thick, red and infrequent urine, and constipation. Opium and nux vomica [a homeopathic medication] have stopped the constipation and probably have acted favorably on the congestion of the eye."[24]

In 1901, Pissarro's seventy-first year, cauterization was continued, as had been done to him for many years. He died 2 years later in 1903.

—— **REFERENCES** ——

1. *Bull Mem Soc Fr Ophtal*, 1884-1926.
2. *Rev Homeop Fr*, 1900-1935.
3. Parenteau D. *Leçons de clinique ophtalmologique*, Doin, Paris, 1881.
4. Parenteau D: *Education de l'oeil et son hygiène*, Pharmacie Centrale Homéopathique, Paris, 1889.
5. Parenteau D: *Thérapeutique homéopathique en ophtalmologie*. Doin, Paris, 1934.
6. Bailly-Herzberg J: *Correspondance de Camille Pissarro*, 5 vols, Valhermeil, Paris, 1988-1992, vol 2, pp. 270-271.
7. Bailly-Herzberg,[6] vol 2, pp. 285-286.
8. Bailly-Herzberg,[6] vol 3, p. 9.
9. Bailly-Herzberg,[6] vol 3, p. 13.
10. Bailly-Herzberg,[6] vol 3, p. 18.
11. Bailly-Herzberg,[6] vol 3, p. 51.
12. Bailly-Herzberg,[6] vol 3, p. 70.
13. Bailly-Herzberg,[6] vol 3, p. 73.
14. Bailly-Herzberg,[6] vol 3, p. 73.
15. Terson A: Sur la destruction du sac au thermo-cautère et son extirpation totale dans les fistules et tumeur lacrimales rebelles, *Arch d'ophtal* 11:224-242, 1891.
16. Terson A: Rapport sur le traitement des affections des voies lacrimales, *Bull Mem Soc Fr Ophtal* 9:3-36, 1891.
17. Toti A: Nuovo metodo conservatore di cura radicale delle suppurazioni croniche del saco lacrimale (dacriocistorinostomia) *La clinica moderna* 10:385-387, 1904.
18. Bailly-Herzberg,[6] vol 3, pp. 74-75.
19. Bailly-Herzberg,[6] vol 3, p. 106.
20. Bailly-Herzberg,[6] vol 4, p. 229.
21. Bailly-Herzberg,[6] vol 4, p. 409.
22. Bailly-Herzberg,[6] vol 4, p. 418.
23. Bailly-Herzberg,[6] vol 5, p. 65.
24. Bailly-Herzberg,[6] vol 5, p. 118.

Chapter Seventeen

THE BLINDNESS OF EDGAR DEGAS

James G. Ravin and Christie Kenyon

The French Impressionist Edgar Degas (1834-1917) (Fig. 17-1) suffered from chronic eye disease. This was a progressive, irreversible loss of vision that became severe in 1870, when he was only 36 years old. The records of the ophthalmologists who are believed to have treated Degas no longer exist. Except for his correspondence and the memoirs of his friends, the only other primary sources of information are the works of art he made. This creates a challenge to those interested in the effects of eye disease on a visual artist. An evaluation of Degas' therapy, considered in light of ophthalmological knowledge in the late nineteenth century, yields some insights into his disability and its effects on his work.

EVOLUTION OF THE OCULAR PROBLEM

Degas' visual problem was present by 1870. He was 36 that year and had enlisted in the National Guard during the Franco-Prussian War. Many years later, Degas wrote that at that time he could not see a rifle target with his right eye.[1] He blamed the loss of vision on the exposure to the elements he suffered as a sentinel during the siege of Paris.[2]

Degas discussed his eyesight in 1871 with his friend and colleague, the English painter Walter Sickert. He described the effect of bright sunlight on his eyes, while attempting to paint outdoors. "I have just had and still have a spot of weakness

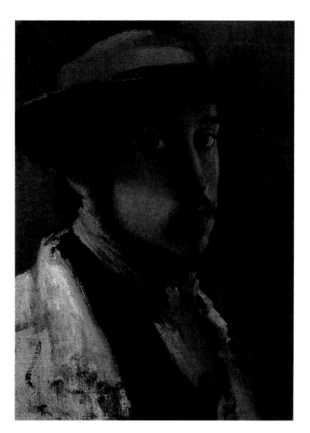

and trouble in my eyes. It caught me at Chatou, by the edge of the water in full sunlight, while I was doing a watercolor, and it made me lose nearly three weeks, being unable to read or go out much, trembling all the while lest I should remain like that."[3] Degas felt that his problems were due to cold weather and to sunlight. The fact that he did not paint outdoors, unlike many of his fellow Impressionists, may have been due to experiences such as this.

In 1873 Degas traveled to New Orleans to visit relatives on his mother's side. In a letter sent back to France, he complained of the intensity of the sunlight in Louisiana. Degas had never been that far south before. "The light is so strong that I have not yet been able to do anything on the river. My eyes are so greatly in need of care that I scarcely take any risk with them at all. A few family portraits will be the sum total of my efforts."[4] Few works from this voyage exist and all are interior scenes. They contain occasional references to the outdoors, indicated by streaks of white paint, perhaps signifying Degas' sensitivity to light. The only completed painting from the trip is *Portraits in an Office*, which was created in his studio from sketches made on site. This became Degas' usual method of working.

During the sojourn to Louisiana, Degas developed a close friendship with his sister-in-law, who also happened to be his first cousin, Estelle Musson de Gas (Fig. 17-2). She was the wife of his brother René. The importance of their relationship goes beyond their blood and marital relationships. Estelle suffered from a progressive eye disease. At that time it was called ophthalmia, a nonspecific and now obsolete term. At age 25 she lost all useful vision in her left eye. The situation deteriorated, so that by age 32 she was blind in both eyes. The parallels of his situation to the more extreme case of his cousin could not have escaped Degas' attention. In fact, his medical history bears a striking similarity to hers. Both suffered severe loss of vision in each eye, with one eye preceding the other by a few years. Edgar's portraits of Estelle, as well as his letters home, reveal a great deal of sympathy for

ter was first described by Jonathan Hutchinson in 1875 as "central chorio-retinal disease in senile persons."[16] Denis said Degas went to the sisters of Saint Germain for care of his eyes after consulting his oculist. This is not surprising, considering the fact that no nineteenth-century oculist had any effective form of therapy available to treat retinal degeneration.

Several pairs of Degas' glasses are in the collection of the Museé d'Orsay in Paris.[17] The lenses vary from no power to a mild myopic astigmatism. The first pair is a pince-nez with no power to the lenses. The lenses are tinted neutral gray, which blocks out about 85% of the incoming light. This pair of glasses appears in an 1876 portrait of Degas by Desboutin and was probably an early form of his treatment. The second pair is a pince-nez tinted slightly more blue than the first pair. The lenses have a mild myopic and astigmatic correction (right eye, plano − 1.00 × 45 degrees; left eye, plano − 1.00 × 135 degrees). The axis is difficult to determine, since the frame of a pince-nez has no fixed position. The third pair is a deeply tinted pair of spectacles with temples. The power of each lens is −1.50 diopters. Photographs of Degas taken from 1890-1900 show him wearing glasses which may have been these. The mild amount of myopia indicates that he should have been able to read most print without glasses if his retinas functioned normally. The fourth pair is the stenopeic spectacle prescription described above. The right side of these spectacles has an occluder for the eye that was severely damaged after 1870. Landolt may have been trying to keep stray light out of Degas' right eye, reduce glare, and discomfort. The left side of these spectacles is a metallic stenopeic slit. This blocks out all rays except those that can enter the slit, 1½ × 15 millimeters in length, set at an axis of 160 degrees. Slits of this type have been used for centuries to reduce light exposure in arctic and desert regions, where intense direct and reflected light can cause extreme visual discomfort. The axis of the stenopeic slit approximates the axis of Degas' astigmatism.

DIAGNOSIS

Degas felt the loss of useful sight in his right eye was related to the cold damp weather he had experienced during the Franco-Prussian War. He felt it was exacerbated by the harsh sunlight of Louisiana. He suffered no known neurologic deficit or other major health problems until very late in his long and productive life. His deficit must have been ocular rather than neurologic in origin. The treatment he received is consistent with this.

He must have retained some sight in the right eye for many decades after his initial complaint in 1870. His eyes remained straight. Photographs of the artist show no evidence of deviation of his eyes. If he had total loss of vision in the right eye, some deviation of that eye would have been likely to have followed. (One exception is an etching of Degas created by his friend Tissot in 1860. It displays an apparent outward deviation of the eyes. But this is probably just a means of expressing emotion, a dreamy and melancholy interpretation of the young Degas. The prominent eyes with droopy lids portrayed by Tissot probably do not reveal an ocular problem since Degas' portraits of his own relatives show the same traits.) The fact that Degas' eyes remained straight, which is evident in photographs taken late in his life, indicates that he retained peripheral fusion, the ability to combine the peripheral visual fields of the two eyes into a single coherent image.

Another reason to conclude that Degas retained some vision in his right eye is based on the fact that his right eye was treated with an occlusive lens in 1893 by Landolt. If Degas had no vision in that eye, he certainly would not have needed an occluder. Degas may have told Landolt that the remaining vision in his poorer seeing right eye was making it difficult for the left eye to see.

Some commentators have suggested that Degas suffered from corneal disease or from uveitis.[17] However, there is no evidence that Degas experienced any externally visible sign of disease of the anterior segments of his eyes. Certainly his friends, physicians, or Degas himself would have noticed overt signs. Diagnosis of a disease of the posterior segment of the eye was often difficult during the late nineteenth century. Mydriatic drops were not always used to dilate the pupil for examination and ophthalmoscopes were crude by today's standards. Landolt was not an expert in retinal disease, despite his wide fame. The sections of his textbook on ophthalmology concerning retinal disease were written by his coauthor, de Wecker, not by Landolt.[18] Degas' close friend and biographer, Halevy, questioned, "What was the true nature of Degas' problem? The oculists seem not to have understood it."[2] It is likely that the abnormality of Degas' eyes was a subtle one, not easily identified by the methods available a century ago.

The brief remembrance of the artist Maurice Denis, that Degas suffered from an untreatable chorioretinitis, is the most specific bit of information available.[8] We have not found reference to this important statement in any other description of Degas, but it clearly points toward the conclusion that Degas suffered from a retinal disease. It may have been infectious, degenerative, or familial in nature. An infectious cause, such as tuberculosis, is one possibility, with scarring involving the right macular more than the left. An hereditary macular degeneration is another. The fact that his first cousin, Estelle Musson de Gas, had similar findings makes a familial form of macular degeneration an interesting possibility. However, the hereditary pattern was not dominant, since no one else is known to have been affected, and it would have been very bad luck for both Edgar and Estelle to have had the same recessive condition.

Degas complained of sensitivity to light. Some individuals who suffer from retinal disease give this symptom and may require an extended period of time to recover from stimulation of their retinas by bright light.[19] Retinal disease could thus have given Degas difficulty in painting outdoors. While inflammation of the anterior segment of the eye can also produce light sensitivity, there is no indication that Degas was treated for this type of problem. Landolt's therapy for corneal disease included topical therapy, even surgery, and subconjunctival injections, but there is no evidence that Degas underwent any of these measures. Landolt's therapeutic program for Degas matches his therapy for retinal disease. Landolt advocated bed rest, avoidance of strong light, and use of tinted lenses for retinal problems.[20]

The fact that Degas encountered difficulty in distinguishing colors[7] supports the concept that he had retinal disease. Color vision abnormalities are common in central retinal disease, but not in corneal disease. Patients with macular disease often require greater color saturation to make up for the washed out appearance of color.[21,22] The intense colors of Degas' late works may have been due, at least in part, to his eye disease. Blue cones are concentrated in the macula, and individuals with central retinal disease frequently have a blue color deficiency. Artists with color vision defects tend to avoid using colors that give them difficulty. It is interesting to note the predominance of red and relative lack of blue in Degas' late works.

Degas' late works show a loss of form when compared with his earlier works. Lanthony has shown how Degas' cross-hatchings can be likened to contrast sensitivity (spatial frequency) testing.[23] His cross-hatchings became much broader and more widely separated as he aged. The change in cross-hatchings correlates with Degas' reduction in vision. Degas' experimentation with sculpture, photography, pastels, and monotypes were probably attempts to explore media better suited to his limited sight than was painting in oil. These media were simpler for him to use than the more complex oil paintings he was used to creating. Oils dry at a much slower rate, and he had the problem of a wet canvas to deal with. This problem did not exist with the other media.

Sickert's comment about Degas' blind spot strongly supports a diagnosis of central retinal disease. Central visual loss is, of course, characteristic of disease involving this area. Degas' complaint that he could only see around the spot at which he was looking and not the spot itself, indicated that he retained peripheral vision during his disability. All commentators on Degas' vision have assumed this refers to Degas' left eye, since the right eye saw next to nothing. The stenopeic spectacles prescribed by Landolt would not have been effective under circumstances of central visual loss. The stenopeic slit would have reduced glare, but would also have made images dark by reducing the amount of light reaching areas of his retina that still worked. A magnifying glass, which Degas found helpful until his vision deteriorated too severely, would have been useful by a mechanism different to that of a stenopeic slit. The magnified image would extend to the portion of the retina that functioned normally. It is no surprise that Degas found a magnifying glass helpful and a stenopeic slit of no use.

Some individuals have suggested that Degas exaggerated his visual problems in order to gain sympathy from his friends or to forestall social situations which he found uncomfortable. The art dealer Ambrose Vollard wrote that "Degas used to pretend to be more blind than he was in order to not recognize people he wanted to avoid." Vollard also wrote that Degas used his deteriorating eyesight as an excuse for not attending art exhibitions with his friends, exclaiming, " 'My eyes! My poor eyes!' Immediately after such a refusal Degas took out his watch and said, without the slightest hesitation, 'It's a quarter past two.' "[24] While there may be some psychological basis for Degas' behavior, this incident can be explained on physical grounds. The fine details of a person's face or a painting would not have been clear to an artist affected by central retinal disease, since the portion of the retina concerned with fine details would not function properly. A watch face with large, dark hands in marked contrast to a lightly colored background would have been easily seen, particularly if held close to the eyes. The image of this watch would be spread out broadly on the retina and not require the fine acuity of the macular region. Undoubtedly, Degas would have had a watch with large hands.

OTHER OPINIONS

In 1965 the art historian Quentin Bell wrote that "the symptoms of his malady suggest, to an expert, the development of senile macular degeneration."[25] Bell consulted a physician for help but he gave no further information. We agree that macular damage is a reasonable diagnosis but would delete the word "senile." Degas was not senile in 1870, when his symptoms became apparent. He was only 36 years old.

The ophthalmologist P.D. Trevor-Roper published his book on eye disease of artists in 1970. He wrote, "Degas was highly myopic, and wore heavy glasses during his adult life."[26] He attributed the loss of central vision in Degas' right eye to the retinal degeneration of high myopia. Trevor-Roper was undoubtedly unaware of the artist's glasses, which show that Degas was only mildly nearsighted. Degas' paintings also give evidence against high myopia. Details are just as indistinct in the foreground as in the background of most of Degas' canvases. In the revised edition of his text (1988), Trevor-Roper changed his opinion. He wrote that Degas "certainly had damage to the macula (the central patch of the retina), which could well be a degenerative change, either from a dystrophy, a sequel to his myopia, or even to an iridochoroiditis."[27] On the basis of Landolt's stenopeic spectacles, Trevor-Roper assumed the artist also suffered from irregular astigmatism. However, Landolt's text indicates stenopeic slits were used for diseases other than irregular astigmatism.

The art historian Richard Kendall published a study of Degas' vision in 1988.[28] He contacted Trevor-Roper and accepted his diagnosis of corneal disease. We have difficulty in accepting this in the absence of substantiating medical records or photographs. We agree with Kendall's findings that the vision in Degas' right eye was nearly, but not totally, lost after 1870, and that sensitivity to light and a central scotoma existed in his left eye. Kendall added two diagnoses which give us difficulty. He wrote Degas was amblyopic in his right eye secondary to an exotropia. An abundance of photographs of the artist exist. None shows a convincing exotropia. Since Degas' ocular problem originated about 1870, when he was 36, it could not have begun in childhood and could not include amblyopia. Kendall accepted the diagnosis of retinal disease in the left eye, which is reasonable to us.

Philippe Lanthony, a French ophthalmologist and expert in color vision, published his views in 1990.[17] Ever cautious, he feels any diagnosis can only be provisional and that a corneal abnormality or an iridochoroiditis are the most likely possibilities.

IMPACT ON HIS CREATIONS

Degas never specifically described the impact of his disability on his art. He referred only to his symptoms, such as his scotoma. His works themselves reveal Degas' adaptation to his visual disturbance in ways that written documents have not. Degas' adjustments to his limitation are found in the applications of his art and in his choice of subject matter. They mark his art as original and deeply personal. Although affected by a progressive eye disease, Degas developed a new sense of vision that enabled him to express his experiences.

Degas began to adjust to his limited sight soon after the onset of his problem in the early 1870s. He explored alternatives to the complex process of oil painting. He experimented with many other media—sculpture, photography, monotypes, and, as the disease progressed, pastel, while working less and less with oils. He found sculpture (Fig. 17-3) and pastel, in particular, to be easier approaches to the themes he was interested in exploring. He could work quickly and broadly in these media, without the concerns of mixing colors on a palette or waiting for the oils to dry in order to revise his efforts.

Since several factors may have contributed to the stylistic changes in Degas' late works, including a conscious simplification of his compositions as well as failing eyesight, the relative contribution of each is difficult to determine. However, there is no question that his sense of artistic form remained good. This did not require precise visual acuity. It is interesting to compare three of his works based on the same theme, the female nude seen from behind (Figs. 17-4, 17-5, and 17-6). These compositions were created at approximately 5- to 10-year intervals, from c. 1890 to c. 1905. Over this 20-year period, the lines of color became more coarse and more widely separated, and the shading became diminished. One critic who visited Degas at his studio in 1907 described his work on a pastel: "The execution was a bit summary like everything currently done by this man, whose eyes are becoming worse each day. But what vigorous and magnificent drawing!"[29]

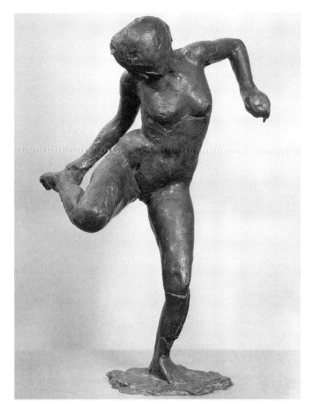

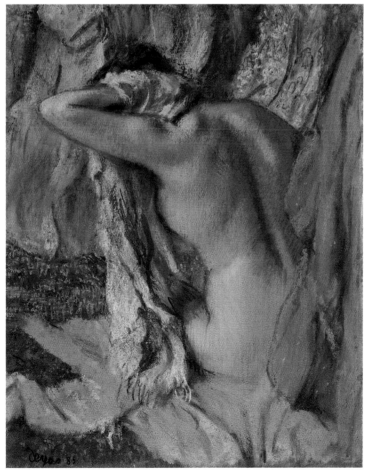

FIGURE 17-4

Degas. *After the Bath.*

Pastel on paper, c. 1890-1895 (dated in error by another hand: 1885). *(The Norton Simon Foundation, Pasadena, Calif.)*

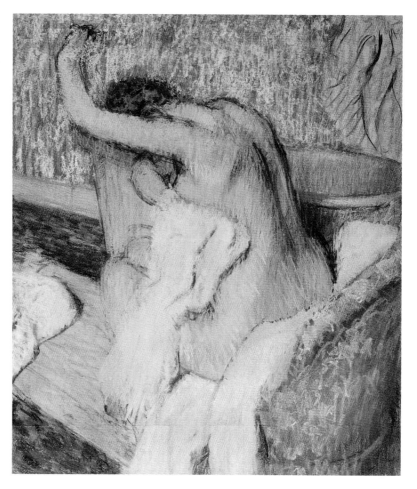

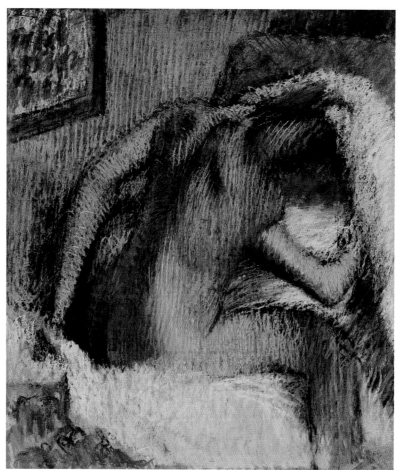

Degas' way of seeing has become a modern point of view. If modern life includes adjusting to the chopped up fragments of our visual experience, then Degas' personal and professional history make him an excellent spokesman for this experience. Degas' visual problems certainly contributed to the way he interpreted the world. He would not have been the same artist if he had normal sight. In the case of this man, visual limitations have created, for the viewer, a liberating experience.

─── REFERENCES ───

1. Blance JE: *Propos de Peinture: De David à Degas*, E. Paul, Paris, 1919, p. 286.
2. Halevy D: *My Friend Degas*, Wesleyan University Press, Middletown, Conn., 1964, p. 22.
3. Guerin M: *Degas Letters*, Cassirer, Oxford, England, 1947, p. 12.
4. Guerin,[3] p. 25.
5. Guerin,[3] p. 34.
6. Sickert W: Degas, *Burlington Magazine* 43:308, 1923.
7. Michel A: Degas et son modèle, *Mercure de France* 131:632, 1919.
8. Barazetti S: Souvenirs de Maurice Denis, *Beaux-arts* 219:D, 1937.
9. Reff J: *The Notebooks of Edgar Degas*, Oxford University Press, Oxford, England, 1976, p. 119.
10. Guerin,[3] p. 39.
11. Reff J: *The Notebooks of Edgar Degas*, Oxford University Press, Oxford, England, 1976, p. 127.
12. Warlomont E: Necrologie, Maurice Perrin, *Ann. d'Ocul* 102:154-156, 1889.
13. Guerin,[3] pp. 184-185.
14. Liebreich R: Turner and Mulready—On the effect of certain faults of vision on painting, with especial reference to their works, *Notices Proc Royal Inst* 6:450-463, 1872.
15. Ravin JG: From Von Graefe's clinic to the Ecole des Beaux-Arts. The meteoric career of Richard Liebreich, *Surv Ophthalmol* 37:221-228, 1992.
16. Gartner S, Henkind P: Aging and degeneration of the human macula, *Br J Ophthalmol* 65:23-28, 1981.
17. Lanthony P: La malvision d'Edgar Degas, *Médecine et hygiène* 48:2382-2401, 1990.
18. de Wecker L, Landolt E: *Traité complet d'ophtalmologie*, 4 vols, Delahaye et Lecrosnier, Paris, 1880-1889.
19. Wu G, et al: Macular photostress test in diabetic retinopathy and age-related macular degeneration, *Arch Ophthalmol* 108:1556-1558, 1990.
20. Landolt E. Gygax P: *Vade Mecum of Ophthalmological Therapeutics*, Lippincott, Philadelphia, 1898, pp. 21, 40-42, 59, 113-117.
21. Fine AM et al: Earliest symptoms caused by neovascular membranes in the macula, *Arch Ophthalmol* 104:513-514, 1986.
22. Alvarez SL, King-Smith PE, Bhargava SK: Spectral thresholds in macular degeneration, *Br J Ophthalmol* 67:508-511, 1983.
23. Lanthony P: Degas et la fréquence spatiale, *Bull Soc Opht Fr* 91:605-611, 1991.
24. Vollard A: *Degas: An Intimate Portrait*, Crown, New York, 1937, p. 22.
25. Bell Q: *Le Viol*, University Press, Newcastle upon Tyne, 1965, n.p.
26. Trevor-Roper PD: *The World through Blunted Sight*, Bobbs-Merrill, Indianapolis, Ind., 1970, pp. 33-34.
27. Trevor-Roper PD: *The World through Blunted Sight*, rev ed, Penguin, London, 1988, p. 39.
28. Kendall R: Degas and the contingency of vision, *Burlington Magazine*, 130:180-197, 1988.
29. Moreau-Nelaton E: Deux heures avec Monsieur Degas. In Lemoisne PA (ed): *Degas et son Oeuvre*, P Braume et CM de Hauke, Paris, 1946, pp. 257-261, n. 218.

Chapter Eighteen

MUNCH AND VISIONS FROM WITHIN THE EYE

Michael F. Marmor

The Norwegian painter Edvard Munch (1863-1944) is famous for his haunting images that probe psychological themes such as love and death. His expressionistic canvases in striking colors, done at the turn of the century, influenced the development of German Expressionism and predated Fauvism (Fig. 18-1). His most famous image is *The Scream* in which stark perspective and a brilliant red sky heighten the sense of mystery and terror. Munch painted throughout his long life (he died in 1944 at the age of 80), but his work was interrupted in 1930 by hemorrhaging in his right eye. As his sight recovered, he made a remarkable series of sketches and pictures showing how the world appeared through the diseased eye.[1] In some of these he drew the debris within the eye, while in others he revealed his aesthetic or emotional response to the disease.

Munch was born on December 12, 1863. His father, a physician, was a strict and religious man who could never quite rationalize the death of Munch's mother from tuberculosis when he was only 5.[2] Death struck the household again 10 years later, when Munch's beloved older sister, Sophie, also died of tuberculosis. The teenaged Edvard had watched his sister waste away from the disease, and the apparent failure of God to avert this disaster contributed to Munch's ultimate rejection of religion and his move toward a Bohemian lifestyle. In his artistic work, he often incorporated images of death intermingled with visions of love and sex. He said of his haunting but sensuous *Madonna* (Fig. 18-2) "She is full of

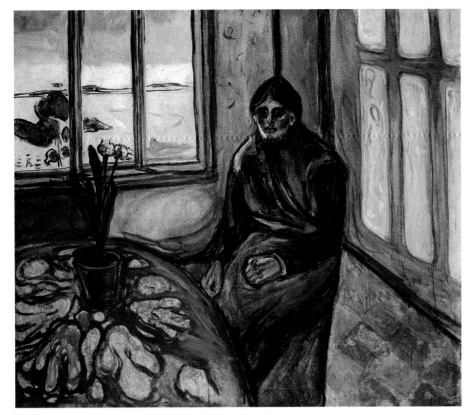

FIGURE 18-1
Munch. *Melancholy (Laura).*
Oil, 1899. Laura is Munch's sister,
who was institutionalized for
mental illness. *(© The Munch
Museum, Olso/The Munch- Ellingsen
Group/Artists Rights Society 1996.)*

the world's beauty and pain" because "death shakes hands with life."[3] Munch had shown a talent for art as a child, and he chose painting as a career much to the consternation of his father. He soon developed an individual style, influenced in part by a visit to Paris in 1885 in which he saw the revolutionary changes in contemporary French art as the era of Impressionism began. In his most productive years, the decades before and after the turn of the century, he lived mainly in Berlin and Paris, and attained international stature as an important artist. However, he suffered a nervous breakdown in 1908, and in 1910 he moved back to Norway permanently where he continued to paint in Ekely (near Oslo) until his death.

Munch was considered a somewhat sickly child, but he outlived all but one of his three siblings. Little is known of his medical history, and he has not been reported to have had any major disorders or disabilities. His left eye was apparently weak for much of his adult life, but the origin or nature of this disability is unknown. He was punched in a fight in 1904, but there is no record of whether this accounts for the poor vision in the left eye.[4] This disability in the left eye did not seriously affect Munch until May 1930 when at the age of 67 he suffered an intraocular hemorrhage in the right eye. His vision was now poor in both eyes, and he was unable to draw or paint for several months until the hemorrhage began to clear. Throughout August and September of 1930 Munch documented what he saw through the diseased right eye in a series of drawings and paintings. They show not only the resolution of an intraocular hemorrhage but also how these changing visual perceptions became integrated into Munch's view of life and art.

The nature of this hemorrhage is unknown. Munch was followed by one of the preeminent eye specialists of the time in Oslo, Professor Johan Raeder, but records of Munch's examinations appear to be lost. Raeder advised Munch to stay at strict rest so that his eye would heal and even gave Munch the following note

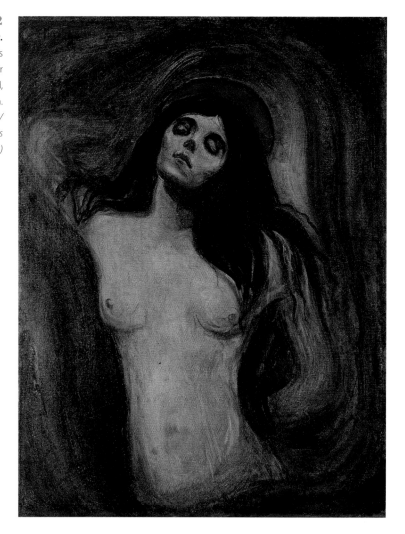

to ward off would-be visitors: "Herr painter Edvard Munch suffers from an acute eye disease caused by a long-standing overexertion. He needs complete bodily and mental rest for a long period of time. Any disturbance, oral, written, by telephone or by telegraph, is to be entirely avoided."[5] A letter by Raeder indicates that Munch had a similar hemorrhage in his left eye in 1938.[6]

It is perhaps ironic that one of Munch's friends and patrons in Germany, Max Linde, was a prominent ophthalmologist. Linde was an avid art collector who bought his first Munch painting in 1902, and he remained in contact with Munch until his death in 1940. However, there is no record that Munch corresponded with Linde about his ocular hemorrhages.

One image that Munch drew during this period of ocular convalescence was a set of concentric circles, sometimes colored vividly (Fig. 18-3). None of these drawings is explicitly labeled, but they resemble the aura about bright lights in a mist or fog, and one may guess that they represent a view through his resolving hemorrhage, possibly while looking toward an electric light or the sun. (Some of the drawings made during his convalescence have been annotated "electric light" or "sunshine.")[7] It is interesting that the colors in these pictures show no consistent order and do not follow the rainbow; some of these drawings are blue on the inside and red on the outside (as those in Fig. 18-3), while others show the reverse. Munch must have been intrigued by these patterns of light and color that appeared in his eye, even if they were signs of an unpleasant reality of disease.

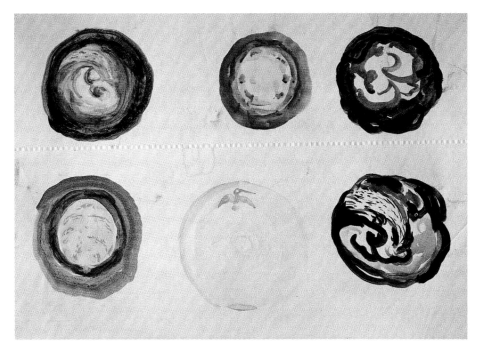

FIGURE **18-3**

Munch. Watercolor, 1930. Circular patterns illustrating his perceptions through vitreous hemorrhage. The colored circles may represent an effect from the sun on an electric light. The middle image of bottom row shows a more shadowy pattern with a branched bird's head figure near the top (T2166).

(© The Munch Museum, Olso/The Munch-Ellingsen Group/Artists Rights Society 1996.)

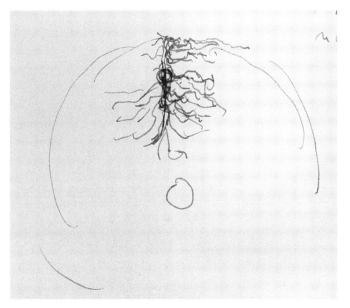

FIGURE **18-4**

Munch. Drawing, 1930. Image of his branched intraocular debris. Subjectively, these wispy patterns reminded him of a bird (see Figs. 18-3, 18-8, and 18-9 [T2136].)

(© The Munch Museum, Oslo/The Munch-Ellingsen Group/Artists Rights Society 1996.)

Munch also drew a number of sketches of the dense but shadowy blind spot in his vision as the blood began to absorb. In some of these sketches, the shadow from the blood is quite opaque and has the vague shape of a skull or of an inverted heart. In others, the obscuration was more tenuous and appeared as a circular haze with a dense branched figure at its upper edge (Figs. 18-4; see also Fig. 18-3). In one of these drawings, Munch drew an arrow to show that his visual fixation point was near the top of the dark shadow created by the blood; and when Munch superimposed the blind spot shadow over sketches of his room, it appeared in the lower part of the scene. This is rather intriguing, in terms of speculation (see below) about possible causes for the hemorrhage.

Munch viewed his resolving eye problem with very precise clinical interest. Some of his sketches of the shadows in his eye were accompanied with notes

FIGURE **18-5**
Munch. Drawing, 1930.
Sketch of letters broken up by
his blind spot (T2149).
*(© The Munch Museum, Oslo/The
Munch-Ellingsen Group/Artists Rights
Society 1996.)*

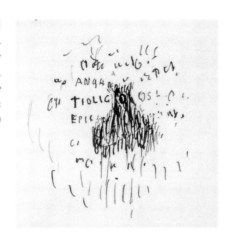

FIGURE **18-6**
Munch. Drawing, 1930.
Intraocular shadow, drawn
over a grid, perhaps as a means of
following the size and shape of his
blind spot over time (T2140).
*(© The Munch Museum, Oslo/The
Munch-Ellingsen Group/Artists Rights
Society 1996.)*

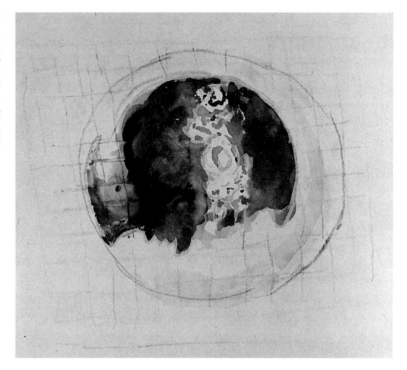

indicating the exact distance of the paper from his face, and the conditions of observation. For example, he drew some letters, partially obscured by his blind spot (Fig. 18-5), along with the notation "In the shadow of full sunshine after the eye has been covered, reading distance, spectacle lens #5."[8] Another sketch is annotated "Bedroom, electric light, no glasses, one-half meter."[9] He even superimposed a grid of lines over some of the drawings to more accurately show and follow the blind spot (Fig. 18-6). This simple idea was in fact a most perceptive innovation and was well ahead of medical practice at the time. We do not know, of course, whether the grid was Munch's idea or had been suggested by Dr. Raeder, but this quantitative method of charting his visual progress was consistent with Munch's scientific approach to optical issues and photography.

Munch's technique of self-examination, with a grid to document the blind spots, anticipated by 17 years the publication by Marc Amsler of Switzerland of printed grids to be used by patients with macular degeneration as a means of self-plotting and recognizing changes in their disease.[10] It is inherently difficult to plot the central visual field when acuity is poor, because subjects have trouble fixat-

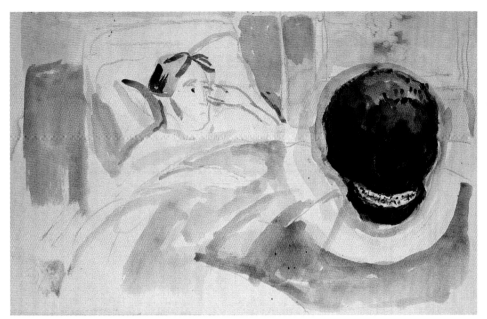

FIGURE **18-7**

Munch. Watercolor and pastel, 1930. Self-portrait in bed, again checking his vision in the right eye. The ominous dark spot from the hemorrhage looms as a death's head over the foot of his bed (T2157). *(© The Munch Museum, Oslo/The Munch-Ellingsen Group/Artists Rights Society 1996.)*

ing with a stable gaze. In the first half of the century, a number of devices were invented to minimize this problem but they were rather complicated.[11,12] For example, one instrument separated the images of the eyes with colored filters so that targets of complementary colors could be used to simultaneously provide a fixation spot in one eye and testing targets for the other. Another method used printed grids that were placed in a stereoscope so that both eyes could help to fixate while the examiner moved tiny targets on the end of a needlelike holder. What Munch—and later Amsler—recognized is that even people with poor vision can orient their gaze quite well within the outline of a square grid and thus can draw the area of their own blind spots. These self-drawn plots are far easier to obtain and quite accurate, and Amsler grids are now widely used in ophthalmology. Munch's grids were not published, of course, and I doubt that Dr. Amsler in Switzerland was aware of Munch's private sketches in Norway.

Munch likened the small dark spot at the top of the shadow (see Figs. 18-3 and 18-4), which had a beaklike extension, to the head of a bird.[1,13] Viewed in this manner, the bulk of the shadow appeared like large and ominous wings (see Fig. 18-6). This "bird" was an image that he would follow over time, writing at one point that "the distance between the bird's beak and the new beak beneath seems longer—I can make out two letters while earlier just one—the bird's neck seems longer—I am clearing up on the left side."[14]

As the major opacity in his eye cleared, he was left with smaller fragments of debris that floated within his eye. "There are dark spots which show up like small flocks of crows far up when I look at the sky—can they be blood clots which have been resting in the periphery of the damaged circular part—which by a sudden movement or by the effect of sharp light are moved from their origin—when they suddenly disappear it looks as if they fly down to their first place."[15]

The fibrillar bird's head probably represented small amounts of blood or reactive tissue layered into the protein framework of the vitreous gel that fills the back of the eye. Alternatively, parts of the bird may represent a detachment of the vitreous independent of the blood. The vitreous gel tends to shrink and collapse with age, and even in eyes that are fundamentally healthy it frequently pulls away from the back wall of the eye. This is ordinarily a benign event, but strands of the partially collapsed gel will cast shadows on the retina that are visible as

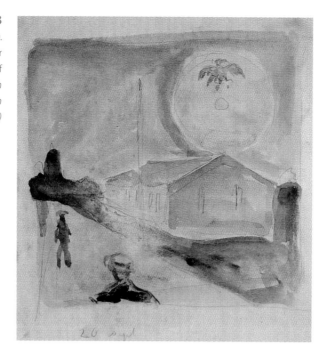

"floaters" and that seem suspended in air when viewed against a bright sky or white wall. The birdlike shape could represent such an area of vitreous condensate lying above the area of the retinal hemorrhage, but we have no record as to whether this floater persisted after 1931 and the image does not appear in Munch's later works.

As his vision improved, Munch made pictures that showed his room, or outdoor scenes, to the extent they would be visible over the residual debris in the eye. Some of these pictures are simply representational and clinical, but others illustrate his past or present emotions or incorporate the shadows artistically rather than objectively. By the time these drawings and paintings were made, Munch was rapidly improving and must have been hopeful of a return to full artistic activity. Yet he had not forgotten that when the hemorrhage first occurred and before the prospects of recovery were evident he was fearful of both blindness and death. For example, in one watercolor (Fig. 18-7), the dense blind spot became a death's head hovering over the foot of his bed, threatening him as he covered his weak left eye to evaluate the view through the right one. On the same day, he also drew an outdoor scene in which a tenuous circular shadow appears high in the sky, perhaps representing an aura about the sun over which is hovering the omnipresent and mysterious floating bird (Fig. 18-8). The blind spot here is painted high in the field of view where it must be symbolic rather than representational. In another picture (Fig. 18-9), he shows himself standing in his room with his hands pressed to his face in a pose similar to that of the famous *Scream*, looking toward the dark shadow bird.

An interesting sideline to these images is the fact that Munch appears in several covering his left eye to evaluate the recovery of the right eye (see Fig. 18-7). Munch painted many self-portraits throughout his long career, and, to make them, he was known to use a mirror, which, by necessity, reverses right and left. In his convalescent works, however, the left eye is always covered correctly; these are not mirror-generated self-portraits but sketches made from memory to illustrate what he saw and what he felt.

Munch's vision apparently cleared further as the year progressed, and birds and blind spots disappeared permanently from his work after 1931. Munch

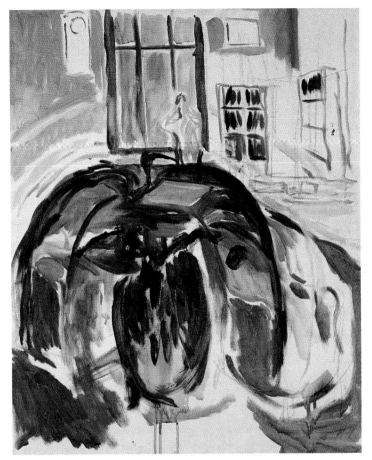

FIGURE 18-9

Munch's room, with a figure (presumably the artist) standing in a pose of fear or anguish, while the sinister bird blots out much of the scene (M341). *(© The Munch Museum, Oslo/The Munch-Ellingsen Group/Artists Rights Society 1996.)*

returned to full-scale painting and continued to work practically up to the time of his death. However, it is perhaps noteworthy that he worked intensively with photography during his convalescence, possibly as a hedge against visual problems that might interfere with painting.

We can only guess about the medical cause of the hemorrhage in Munch's eye. His description of blood clots and debris floating within his field of vision strongly suggest that he hemorrhaged into the interior (vitreous gel) of his eye. At the same time, there is evidence that the source of hemorrhage—and indeed some of the hemorrhage itself—was intraretinal and localized to the macula. For example, as his vision was clearing, the circular shadow he perceived was fixed rather precisely just *below* his center of gaze. If all of the hemorrhage had been free within the vitreous, it would have settled (by gravity) into the lower part of the eye and produced a shadow in the upper part of his vision. Munch's shadow was also rather small relative to the full extent of normal vision, which suggests a local area of bleeding. It is likely that Munch's primary hemorrhagic disease was in his central retina, but some of the blood broke out into the vitreous.

Modern surveys of spontaneous vitreous hemorrhage list diabetic retinopathy, retinal tears, blockage of the retinal veins, contraction of the vitreous gel (posterior vitreous detachment), and retinal detachment as the most common causes.[16] There is no evidence that Munch was diabetic, and he would have been unlikely to have survived 14 more years in those days with good vision and good health. He clearly did not have a retinal detachment, which would have required surgery to restore vision. Small tears in the peripheral retina may cause hemorrhage into the vitreous, but would be unlikely to cause a fixed blind spot close to the center of view. Posterior vitreous detachment was discussed earlier in this chapter as a cause of floaters. The vitreous gel can on rare occasions tear a small vessel as it pulls away from the retina, but the hemorrhages are unlikely to persist or affect vision seriously. Blockage of a branch retinal vein is not a rare event in Munch's age group, and is perhaps the most likely of all the possibilities. Because separate vessels feed the upper and lower halves of the retina, occlusion of a small branch just above the center of the macula will cause a loss of vision below the point of fixation. However, Munch was not known to be hypertensive (a predisposing factor), the blind spot with a vein occlusion is not usually a well-defined circle, and the areas of vascular blockage do not usually recover vision.

Among the less frequent causes of vitreous hemorrhage is age-related macular degeneration. This disorder is the largest cause of visual disability among older Americans (see Chapter 19), but it only rarely causes bleeding into the vitreous and when bleeding occurs the visual prognosis is usually poor. Another rare cause of hemorrhage would be a retinal vascular malformation in the eye, but there is no direct evidence for this diagnosis. We are left with the dilemma of choosing an uncommon manifestation of a common disease, or choosing an uncommon disorder. Neither is satisfying without better supporting evidence—and the issue is moot with respect to Munch's art because he recovered good vision, returned to painting, and remained physically active until the time of his death.

Munch's eye disease was only a brief interlude in his long career, and it occurred long after he produced his most famous works. Although his regular painting was interrupted for nearly a year, his career was not cut short or permanently compromised as with the visual problems that afflicted Monet, Cassatt, Degas, and O'Keefe (see Chapters 14, 15, 17, and 19). Thus, his work from this period affords an interesting glimpse into his method and his mind, under circumstances where we know that his ultimate approach to art was not altered. His sketches and drawings from the period of his illness are in one sense clinical and describe what he saw. And yet, they describe it in the unmistakable style of the artist. Like a subject doing a Rorschach test, Munch shares with us the visions evoked by his intraocular debris, and he incorporates these visions into paintings that are both artistic and poignant. One might argue that in some respects these pictures are no different than any other paintings of places, people, or events in which an artist has invested the scene with his or her own interpretations. The difference here is that part of the scene lies within the eye, and the painter is revealing a landscape that no one else can see.

--- **REFERENCES** ---

1. Eggum A: *Munch and Photography,* Yale University Press, New Haven, Conn., 1989.
2. Heller R: *Munch, His Life and Work,* University of Chicago Press, Chicago, 1984.
3. Notes in Munch Museum, Oslo, inventory number T2782. Quoted in Schneeds UM: *Edvard Munch. The Early Masterpieces,* WW Norton, New York, 1988, p. 70.
4. Eggum A: Personal communication, June 22, 1995.
5. Raeder J: Letter dated May 10, 1930, Munch Museum, Oslo. The same letter was reissued almost word for word on September 27, 1930.
6. Raeder J: Letter dated March 29, 1938, Munch Museum, Oslo.
7. Notes on sketches T2143, T2148, T2165, Munch Museum, Oslo.
8. Sketches and notes T2149, Munch Museum, Oslo.
9. Notes on sketch T2148, Munch Museum, Oslo.
10. Amsler M: L'examen qualitatif de la fonction maculaire, *Ophthalmologica* 114:248-261, 1947.
11. Evans JJ: The field of vision, *The Ophthalmoscope* 9:698-711, 1911.
12. Dubois-Poulsen A: *Le Champ Visuel,* Masson, Paris, 1952.
13. Lanthony P: L'oiseau d'Edvard Munch, *Bull Soc Ophtalmol Fr* 94:555-559, 1994.
14. Notes on T2136, Munch Museum, Oslo.
15. Notes on T2167, Munch Museum, Oslo.
16. Dana M-R, Werner MS, Viana MAG, Shapiro MJ: Spontaneous and traumatic vitreous hemorrhage, *Ophthalmology* 100:1377-1383, 1993.

Chapter Nineteen

THE BLURRED WORLD OF GEORGIA O'KEEFFE

James G. Ravin and Michael F. Marmor

The paintings of Georgia O'Keeffe (1887-1986) are easily recognized. Many of her unique images are oversized and disproportionate to our usual way of seeing. The colors are bright, sometimes very luminous, as was the sun at her home in New Mexico. Her painted edges are often hard, as may be seen in high contrast black-and-white photography. These edges differ from the modulated contours of many old master paintings and with the art school aphorism "there are no lines in nature." However, her sharp edges are balanced by dramatic shading that gives a feeling of three-dimensionality and sensuality to her works.

In her flower paintings, she depicted overly large plants in broad sweeps of color, sometimes creating effects that are close to abstraction. These magnified views make the observer look closely at aspects of the subject which would ordinarily be overlooked, and thus one can find new forms and associations in the blend of shapes and colors. Her landscapes (Fig. 19-1) are characterized by graded colors and overlapping hills that evoke Asian brush paintings and are instantly recognizable as being by O'Keeffe.

Late in her life, O'Keeffe wrote, "Objective painting is not good painting unless it is good in the abstract sense."[1] In this spirit, she often found beauty and joy in simple shapes, such as *Green Lines and Pink* (Fig. 19-2). The shading is luminous and tantalizing, and the abstract forms take on body as if they were real objects. O'Keeffe makes us focus on contrasts of light and dark, even though some of our

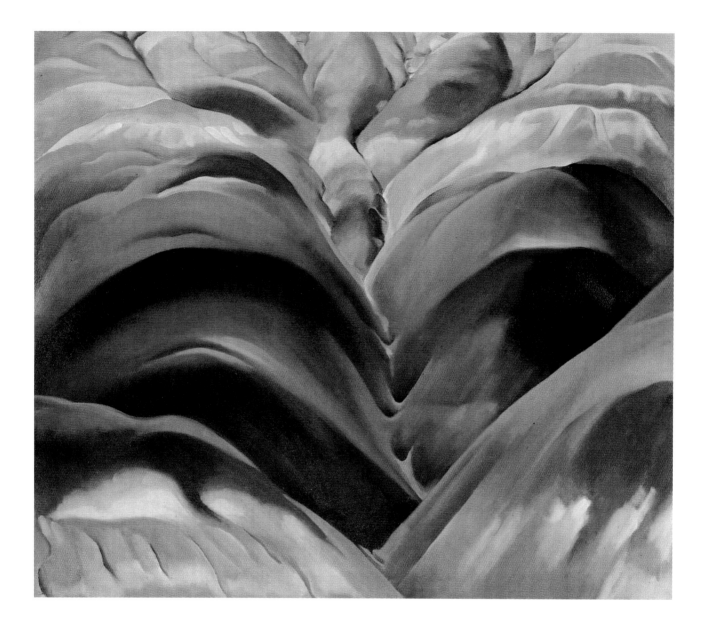

FIGURE 19-1

O'Keeffe. *Black Place #1.*

Oil on canvas, 1944. (© 1996 The
Georgia O'Keeffe Foundation/Artists
Rights Society [ARS], New York. San
Francisco Museum of Modern Art. Gift
of Charlotte Mack.)

perceptions may be illusory. The apparent darkness and lightness of the background is influenced by the Mach bands (see Chapter 6) painted at the lines.

O'Keeffe was fortunate to live into her ninety-ninth year. With advancing age, however, came severe loss of vision due to macular degeneration and a central retinal vein occlusion. These ocular problems were great hardships for her and caused her to make major changes both in her lifestyle and in her approach to art. This artist, who had enjoyed being in control of her destiny, became forced to rely on others for the most basic activities of everyday life. She had been proud of her excellent vision and had come to take it for granted. Except for a brief episode of ocular inflammation associated with an attack of measles in adulthood, her eyesight had always been remarkably good.

For a period of time in her sixth decade, she was an enthusiastic follower of the Bates method of eye exercises.[2] In a book entitled *Perfect Sight without Glasses*, the eccentric Dr. W.H. Bates described his technique of getting rid of the need for spectacles.[3] He claimed that poor eyesight was caused by poor visual habits. One of his exercises includes the dangerous recommendation of fluttering the eyelids

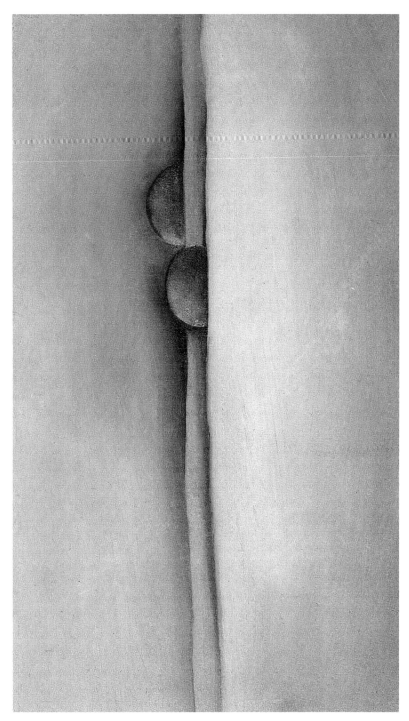

FIGURE   **19-2**
O'Keeffe. *Green Lines and Pink.*
Oil on canvas, 1919. The relative
brightness of the background
changes if one covers the shaded
vertical lines. *(© 1996 The Georgia
O'Keeffe Foundation/Artists Rights
Society [ARS], New York. Photo by:
Malcolm Varon, N.Y.C. © 1996.)*

while looking directly at the sun. It is not known if O'Keeffe performed this specific exercise, but if she did it might have been a factor in the development of her
loss of vision. She may also have been influenced by the British author Aldous
Huxley, whom she knew. He had first tried the Bates method in 1937,[4] and
eventually became such a strong advocate of Bates' unscientific theories that he
wrote a book, *The Art of Seeing*, relating his experiences with the method.[5] He
said that his vision improved so greatly from the exercises that he no longer
needed glasses.

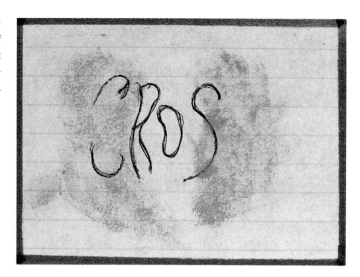

O'Keeffe was obstinate about her vision and refused to wear sunglasses even under the powerful New Mexico sunlight.[2,6] She objected to the distortions of colors that tinted lenses induced. However, excess exposure to sunlight can predispose one to certain types of cataract, and it is thought to be a risk factor in the development of macular degeneration.[7] Epidemiological evidence for the latter is weak, but in experimental situations intense or prolonged light exposure (especially ultraviolet) is damaging to the retina. The strong sunlight of the Southwest may have had something to do with the fact that O'Keeffe developed a severe case of macular degeneration which limited her ability to paint. However, it is probably of greater relevance that she had a family history of this disease, which depends in part on hereditary predisposition. Her maternal grandfather, George Totto, suffered from it. (She had been named Georgia Totto O'Keeffe in his honor.[8])

Macular degeneration is the major cause of visual disability among the elderly in our society. It accounts for more visual loss in individuals over age 55 than any other disorder, including cataracts (since they are curable by surgery). In most people, the process is a slow and indolent degeneration of the central part of the retina (the macula), which can make images hazy, fragmented, and distorted. Fig. 19-3 was drawn by a patient to illustrate how images become distorted and fragmented with central gaps but preserved peripheral vision. As the disease progresses, the central vision becomes worse, and in advanced cases only the peripheral vision remains. In some individuals blood vessels and scar tissue grow into the diseased macula and these fragile new vessels can hemorrhage or leak fluid. Such exudative or "wet" macular degeneration damages vision more quickly and severely. This is the form of the disease that eventually afflicted O'Keeffe.

It is perhaps a commentary on medical progress that whereas presbyopia and cataracts were the most prevalent visual disasters to befall elderly painters before the twentieth century (see Chapters 2 and 5), it was their cure by glasses and modern surgery that exposed the scourge of macular degeneration. The latter was hardly appreciated in ancient times because cataract would be diagnosed if present, there were no instruments to look at the retina, and few people lived long enough to be afflicted. In fact, macular degeneration did not receive much space in the ophthalmologic literature until the latter half of the twentieth century, when increasing life expectancy made late visual loss a more prevalent problem, and the development of ophthalmic cameras, fluorescein angiography, and therapeutic lasers made better diagnostic distinctions and therapy possible. Prevention and cure of this disease is now a major ophthalmologic priority, to preserve not only the productivity of superannuated artists but the visual future of us all.

According to a recent biography of the artist, O'Keeffe first noticed the symptoms of macular degeneration in 1964. She was 77 that year. She "was driving from Ghost Ranch on a brilliantly sunny day when she experienced the shock of her life. As her Buick convertible rounded a curve in the road and the valley narrowed to a patch of greenery along the river, her vision was obscured. It felt, she said later, as if a cloud had entered her eyeballs—and, in a way, it had. She called a friend on the phone. 'My world is blurred!' the artist cried into the receiver. For years, only those very close to the artist knew about her problem."[9] She was examined by her personal physician, Dr. Constance Friess, in autumn 1964 and was diagnosed as having macular degeneration. She came under the care of Frank Constantine, M.D., chairman of the department of ophthalmology at the Manhattan Eye and Ear and Throat Hospital.

Back home in New Mexico, she was the patient of Walter J. Levy, M.D., an ophthalmologist who practiced in Santa Fe. He has written that "this fascinating lady was a patient of mine from 1972 through 1979. She proved to be quite a character. She would arrive unannounced in my waiting room in her nun-like outfit, looking like Queen Victoria, and regally inform my staff that she would be seen momentarily. My other patients seemed to tolerate this intrusion with good humor." Levy continued, "When I first saw her she had a severe exudative maculopathy in the right eye with extensive pigmentary changes and laser retinal scarring surrounding. The left eye had the typical hemorrhagic vascular changes of a vein occlusion"[10] that had occurred in December 1971. She was unfortunate to have had this additional problem in the left eye on top of her macular degeneration. Retinal vein occlusions occur when a vein becomes compressed or thrombosed, causing ischemia and the rupture of many small capillaries within the retina. The end result is usually very poor visual acuity. The condition is not uncommon among the elderly and is often associated with hypertension.

Dr. Levy found her vision to be less than 20/200 in each eye and not improvable with glasses. However she could read very small print (J2 size letters) with a telescopic spectacle. "She tried this," he wrote, "but was too impatient to use it well. I suggested to her that she continue painting with a very broad sweeping technique to allow for her central scotomatous handicap. Through the years on regular visits her condition remained fairly static."[10]

In the mid-1970s, she consulted Glenn O. Dayton, Jr., M.D., a specialist in retinal disease who practiced in Los Angeles. She had been advised to see him by a friend in Santa Fe, New Mexico, whom he had treated with laser photocoagulation for macular degeneration. Dr. Constantine wrote Dr. Dayton and gave him details of O'Keeffe's case. Dr. Dayton has written that he remembered her well. "She was quite elderly with gray hair pulled back in a severe manner, quite alert and not interested in any nonsense. . . . Both maculae were thoroughly destroyed by a degenerative atrophic process with no thought of treatment by any type of modality. Her New York physician had informed her of this and she rather stoically accepted my concurring opinion. I might add she showed little evidence of blindness in her moving about the consultation room or reception area."[11]

She consulted another ophthalmologist in Santa Fe, Tim Knowles, M.D. When he examined her a few years before her death in 1986, she had extensive macular disease.[12] She had also been examined at several other major medical centers in the United States and in England.

One recent biographer of O'Keeffe, Hogrefe, stated: "As her eyesight failed progressively, she became increasingly suspicious and paranoid. One of her friends noted that she was always losing things in this period and accusing other people of stealing them."[13] This unfortunate type of behavior is reminiscent of that of Cassatt and Degas. As these two artists aged and lost vision, both became alien-

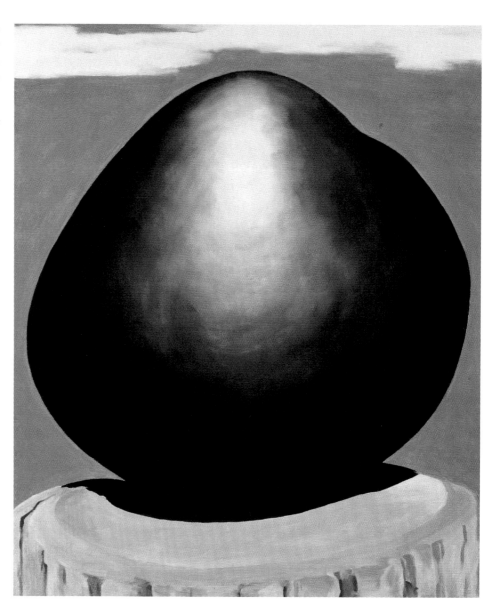

ated from friends with whom they had been very close for years. They became unreasonably suspicious and made sad, erroneous accusations about others.

Hogrefe also wrote: "Like many disabled people, O'Keeffe discovered that her other senses were heightened as she lost her sight."[13] This type of commentary has also been applied to Degas, who turned to sculpture as a more tactile artistic medium when he found it difficult to paint in oils, due to his poor eyesight. Degas, in all likelihood, also suffered from macular dysfunction (see Chapter 17). O'Keeffe and Degas may have become more aware of their other senses, such as touch and hearing, but these senses could not have really improved. Like Degas, O'Keeffe did not give up painting entirely when her vision became severely impaired. Both continued to paint, but less often, and created painted works that have far fewer details than the works they created when their eyesight was good.

Few illustrations of O'Keeffe's late works have been published to date, and those available only hint at the impact of visual loss on her art. The *Black Rock* series occupied O'Keeffe between 1970 and 1971, a time when her vision was failing to critical levels. *Black Rock with Blue Sky and White Clouds,* dated 1971-1972

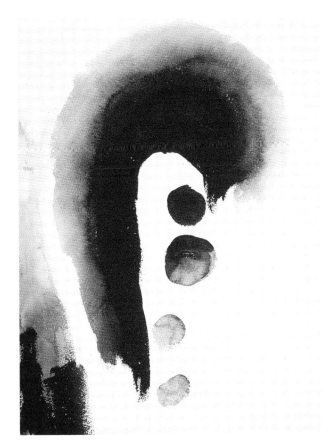

FIGURE   19-5

O'Keeffe. *Red Line with Circle.*

Watercolor on paper, 1977. *(© 1996
The Georgia O'Keeffe Foundation/
Artists Rights Society [ARS], New York.
Private collection. Photo by: Malcolm
Varon, N.Y.C. © 1996.)*

(Fig. 19-4), may be compared with her earlier works in Figs. 19-1 and 19-2. It
shows much less subtlety of shading, and she painted a harsh, pitch black shadow that is devoid of gradation. The focus of the picture on a single natural shape
is as powerful as ever, but the delicacy of shading and contrasts that are so unique
in O'Keeffe's work are missing.

Macular degeneration not only affects visual acuity (i.e., the resolution of
small objects) but also diminishes the critical ability to judge contrast (see Chapter
1). Even without a serious loss of acuity, many elderly individuals have difficulty
recognizing objects at dusk or in dim light. Macular degeneration can also diminish color sense and make adaptation to changing light conditions more difficult.
This type of visual difficulty must have been especially disturbing to an artist like
O'Keeffe, whose style and content were directly dependent on subtle components
of vision. Indeed, one way she recognized visual trouble was dimness rather than
blur: "I'd been to town and was going home. And I thought to myself, well, the
sun is shining, but it looks so grey. I thought that's a little funny, but I didn't pay
any attention to it."[14] It is a tribute to O'Keeffe's will power how long she perse-
vered with her art under these conditions.

Toward 1976 O'Keeffe tried to compensate for her visual loss by having assistants help her paint her canvases. Though her central vision was poor, there were
gaps through which she could see better, and she would use these glimpses of
clarity to direct the choice and application of colors. One of her assistants, John
Poling, described her visual struggles as she tried to demonstrate painting technique: "Bare patches of canvas were overlooked. . . . Sometimes she painted the
same small area twice. . . . then she might continue several inches away, thinking she was where she had left off. . . . I had an odd feeling: her brush movements
should have produced something significantly different from what appeared on

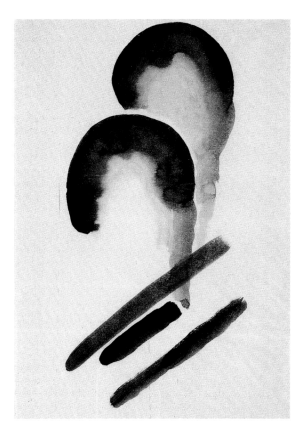

the canvas. I realized she must have made those movements by habit, from memory. Though her motions were sure and those of a master, she could not maneu-
ver or adjust them based on what came through her eyes." On another day Poling
placed a small sliver of charcoal on a black table where it was hard to see.
O'Keeffe "moved toward the black table, scanning its surface. Suddenly and
unerringly she picked up the piece of charcoal. I was surprised. 'It's like there are
little holes in my vision,' she said. 'I can't see straight on very well. But around
the edges are little holes where I can see quite clearly.' "[15]

One of the paintings created with Poling's assistance was published in *Art
News* in the next year, and Poling complained that he was given no credit for it.
O'Keeffe was furious—perhaps more from distress that the world would invade
her privacy and know of her blindness than from jealousy. She told a reporter
that her assistant "was the equivalent of a palette knife. . . . nothing but a tool.
. . . Since the beginning of time, artists have had assistants."[16] It is interesting
that in his reminiscence Poling described clearly the tight artistic control that
O'Keeffe maintained: "The color I mixed wasn't right. She eyed the palette
intently. I made some adjustments. . . . When she thought it seemed right I
began applying it." He even acknowledged that "what we had painted so far
was like the anticipation of some wonderful secret; it was as if O'Keeffe knew
the secret and took pleasure in witholding it from me."[15] This distinction
between an artist, who conceives and understands an image, and a craftsman
who merely realizes it, was accepted in earlier eras when artist's workshops
were common, but modern critics have a fetish for provenance. There is no
question that technical assistance may influence the style or appearance of a
painting, but whether this matters is a judgment that probably should not be
made a priori: we would surely not criticize Matisse for shifting his technique
to paper cutouts when he could no longer paint. However, the issue remains

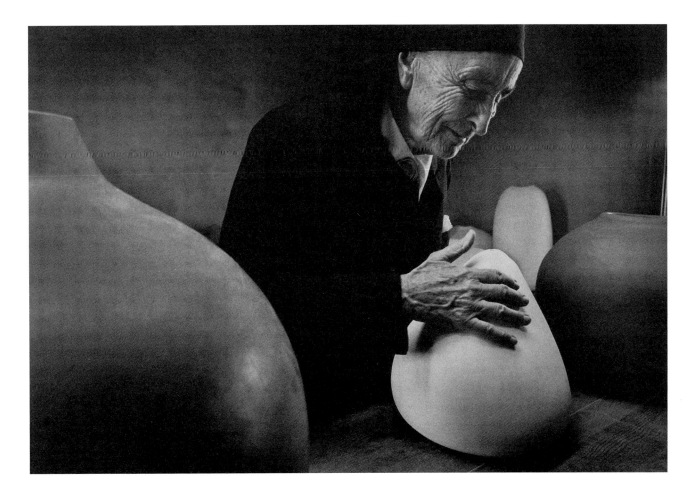

FIGURE   **19-7**
O'Keeffe with Juan Hamilton's pots in the Ghost Ranch studio. Photograph by Dan Budnik. *(© 1996 Dan Budnik.)*

one of consequence where poor vision may prevent the artist from exercising a full degree of aesthetic control.

Whether the criticism of O'Keeffe was justified or not, she was stung by the negative publicity; she ceased using assistants and did no further oil painting. She did produce some late watercolors that are interesting in terms of her artistic development as well as her sight. They have been described as "increasingly simplified,"[17] using saturated colors in discrete single images (Fig. 19-5). One might look at these simple shapes, still powerful in conception but lacking in detail, and argue that they illustrate the limits of her vision. This may be true insofar as she could no longer produce the complex visual effects that had characterized her mature painting, but the forms and execution of these watercolors are in fact a reprise of ideas and techniques that she used while experimenting with abstract shapes during her early formative years (Fig. 19-6).

As Degas turned increasingly to sculpture when his vision diminished, O'Keeffe also turned to a tactile, three-dimensional artistic medium when her vision became poor. For her, this medium was pottery. She was instructed in pottery by Juan Hamilton, a potter who also served as an assistant about her home. For both O'Keeffe and Degas, the preference for a tactile, three-dimensional format was neither total nor new. Both had worked in sculpture before their eyesight became significantly problematic. There is perhaps a resemblance between O'Keeffe judging pots by feel (Fig. 19-7) and the Greek vase painter Euphronios who turned to potting at the age of presbyopia (see Fig. 5-8).

Nonmedical observers of O'Keeffe have given interesting evaluations of her eyesight. One noted that "she wasn't completely blind; she could see shadows.

And there were times when she could see more than at other times, perhaps because of the quality of the light. Sometimes she'd ask me what the moon looked like or ask me about the clouds. Once when we were outside walking she looked up and said, 'Well, I see there are clouds in the sky.' She could see the movement of things and large patterns."[18] Another individual who interviewed her at age 90, in 1977, appeared to be in awe of the artist and clearly overestimated the artist's visual acuity: "I had heard that her eyes were failing, but during this interview I had noticed nothing wrong with them. She is surefooted along narrow paths and precarious bridges, pointing with her cane to all sorts of details in her garden. She looks carefully at her new paintings and watercolors, telling me about them. She also chides me when I am not looking at her. She points out every mountain on the horizon. Her distance vision appears to be perfect. It is the small, closeup thing that she cannot see. And yet, she says, sometimes she can see the tiniest piece of lint on the floor." The most important aspects of this interview are not the writer's judgments about O'Keeffe's visual acuity but the documentation of her continued dedication and her perseverance in spite of her acquired visual deficit: "O'Keeffe says simply, 'I can see what I want to paint. The thing that makes you want to create is still there.'"[19] She remained dedicated until the end of her life.

— REFERENCES —

1. O'Keeffe G: *Georgia O'Keeffe*, Viking Press, New York, 1976, text accompanying fig. 88.
2. Lisle L: *Portrait of an Artist*, Seaview Books, New York, 1980, p. 237.
3. Bates WH: *Perfect Sight without Glasses*, Holt, New York, 1920.
4. Bedford S: *Aldous Huxley*, Carroll and Graf, New York, 1985, p. 366.
5. Huxley A: *The Art of Seeing*, Harper and Row, New York, 1942. Reprinted by Creative Arts Book Co., Berkeley, Calif., 1982.
6. Hogrefe J: *O'Keeffe. The Life of an American Legend*, Bantam Books, New York, 1992, p. 257.
7. Taylor HR et al: Visible light and risks of age-related macular degeneration, *Trans Am Ophthalmol Soc* 88:163-178, 1990.
8. Robinson R: *Georgia O'Keeffe*, Harper and Row, New York, 1989, p. 514.
9. Hogrefe J,[6] p. 229.
10. Levy W: Letter to JG Ravin dated December 18, 1990.
11. Dayton GO Jr: Letter to JG Ravin dated March 4, 1991.
12. Puro GV: Letter to JG Ravin dated January 23, 1991.
13. Hogrefe,[6] p. 298.
14. Warhol A: Georgia O'Keeffe and Juan Hamilton, *Interview* 13:54-55, 1983.
15. Poling J: Painting with Georgia O'Keeffe. In Merrill C and Bradbury E (eds): *From the Faraway Nearby: Georgia O'Keeffe as Icon*, Addison-Wesley, Reading, Mass., 1992, pp. 193-209.
16. Aldrich H: Art assist: Where is credit due? in Castro JG: *The Art and Life of Georgia O'Keeffe*, Crown, New York, 1995, p.176, and Robinson R,[8] pp. 514, 538 (originally published in the *Santa Fe Reporter*, July 31, 1980, p. 5).
17. Haskell B: A critical essay. In O'Keeffe G: *Works on Paper*, Museum of New Mexico Press, Santa Fe, 1985, pp. 1-13.
18. Patten CT, Cardona-Hine A: Days with Georgia, *Art News*, April 1992, p. 109.
19. Klotz ML: Georgia O'Keeffe at 90, *Art News*, December 1977, p. 40.

INDEX